Maria A. Motta da Silva Esser
Fabiana Mamede

Qualified care for women in labour

Maria A. Motta da Silva Esser
Fabiana Mamede

Qualified care for women in labour

The reality of nursing care in the city of Londrina-PR

Imprint

Any brand names and product names mentioned in this book are subject to trademark, brand or patent protection and are trademarks or registered trademarks of their respective holders. The use of brand names, product names, common names, trade names, product descriptions etc. even without a particular marking in this work is in no way to be construed to mean that such names may be regarded as unrestricted in respect of trademark and brand protection legislation and could thus be used by anyone.

Cover image: www.ingimage.com

This book is a translation from the original published under ISBN 978-3-330-76347-0.

Publisher:
Sciencia Scripts
is a trademark of
Dodo Books Indian Ocean Ltd. and OmniScriptum S.R.L publishing group

120 High Road, East Finchley, London, N2 9ED, United Kingdom
Str. Armeneasca 28/1, office 1, Chisinau MD-2012, Republic of Moldova, Europe
Managing Directors: Ieva Konstantinova, Victoria Ursu
info@omniscriptum.com

Printed at: see last page
ISBN: 978-620-8-40536-6

To my family, my mother, Elza, my father, Milton, my brother, Júnior, and my sister-in-law, Cíntia, for their support and intense understanding.
To my husband, Wendel, and my daughter, Bianca, for encouraging me through the most difficult times.

ACKNOWLEDGEMENTS

To God for giving me the strength to complete this dream and for always being present in my life.

To my supervisor Prof Dr Fabiana Villela Mamede, for her friendship, respect, simplicity and dedication. Thank you very much for your guidance and for sharing your research experience.

To Profs. Dr Maria José Clapis and Ana Márcia Spanó Nakano, for their suggestions during my qualifying exam.

To all the teachers of the postgraduate courses; throughout this process, they were attentive, patient, unselfish in their knowledge, sharing knowledge and learning that contributed greatly to my training.

To my friends at Pitágoras College, especially the Director, Marcos Jerônimo Goroski Rambalducci, an example of professionalism, for his recognition, support and constant encouragement for my training.

To my friend Regina Stella Spagnuolo, for always being with me at the best of times and pushing me forward in my teaching career.

To my lifelong friend, Luciane Maria Stahl, for being there for me on this journey.

To the parturients and health professionals who made this study possible by sharing their experiences.

To my friends and all the special people who have been and are part of my life and who have helped me in one way or another to achieve this goal.

SUMMARY

Reducing maternal mortality is one of the health indicators whose main element is quality labour and birth care. The International Confederation of Midwives (ICM) advocates the skills and competences needed to provide quality nursing care throughout the pregnancy and childbirth cycle. <u>Objectives: to</u> characterise the nursing professionals who work in childbirth care and to analyse the essential competences developed by these professionals. <u>Methodology:</u> This is a descriptive study with a quantitative approach, carried out in three maternity hospitals. The study population consisted of 63 nursing professionals (28 nursing assistants, 22 nursing technicians, 8 obstetric nurses and 5 nurses). Through non-participant observation, 92 deliveries were followed up sequentially, during admission, labour and delivery and the immediate postpartum period, in all the institutions surveyed. Descriptive statistics were used to analyse the data. <u>Results</u>: profile of the nursing professionals: all the professionals are female, with an average age of 38.1 years, 68.3% are married or live with a partner and the majority are financially dependent; they work an average of 64.25 hours a week. We observed that the auscultation of the BCF and vaginal touch were incompletely performed, as was the use of the partogram, which was adopted in only one of the institutions. We noted that births attended by obstetric nurses are registered as medical procedures, contrary to Brazilian legislation. <u>Conclusion</u>: We observed that there are differences in the quality of nursing care provided in the institutions participating in this study. Therefore, we cannot say that the care provided in the municipality complies with WHO and Ministry of Health standards regarding the quality of care provided. Many essential skills for labour and delivery care are not developed. Institutions need incentives to implement actions based on up-to-date evidence.

Keywords: nursing care, professional competences, nursing team, obstetric nursing.

SUMMARY

CHAPTER 1

INTRODUCTION

1.1 Presentation

The proposal for this study is part of an extensive project on the "Mapping of Obstetrics/Parole Services in the Americas", coordinated by the Pan American Health Organisation (PAHO), the purpose of which is to gather information on obstetric services in each participating country, to guide the support that PAHO will provide to countries in the future, in order to promote risk-free maternity care throughout Latin America and the Caribbean. The School of Ribeirão Preto/USP, as a World Health Organisation Collaborating Centre for Research, is a partner in this task force and has taken on the coordination of the research in Brazil.

As an obstetric nurse working in maternity hospitals in the interior of the state of Paraná, I have often come across situations in which nursing care has been fundamental to childbirth care and, from this perspective, I was interested in carrying out this study and seeking out the real role of the professional nurse and the essential competences that the obstetric nursing team must develop. This concern has a wider scope, in the sense that it seeks to build knowledge about the true reality of obstetric nursing care in Latin America.

1.2 Qualified Care for Women in Childbirth

The need for effective measures to combat the extreme risk of death or the condition of living in situations of disability or mutilation among women and their children is proven when we look at a scenario that reveals that every year, from an estimated 120 million pregnancies that occur in the world, approximately 600,000 women between the ages of 15 and 40 die as a result of pregnancy and birth complications. More than 50 million women suffer serious illnesses or disabilities related to the pregnancy-partum-puerperium process, which affect their well-being for the rest of their lives. Similarly, at least 1.2 million newborns die from complications during labour (WHO, 1999; Macdonald & Starrs, 2003).

Maternal mortality estimates developed by the World Health Organisation (WHO), the United Nations Children's Fund (UNICEF) and the United Nations Population Fund (UNFPA) indicate that in 2000, the estimated number of maternal deaths was 529,000 worldwide. The maternal mortality ratio (MMR) is estimated to be around 400 per 100,000 live births worldwide (WHO, 2003).

In developing countries, one woman in 16 may die from complications related to pregnancy and birth, compared to one in 2,800 pregnancies in developed countries. Each death or long-term complication represents an individual tragedy for the woman, her partner, her family and the community (WHO, 2004).

In Brazil, high maternal mortality rates are a cause for concern for health authorities at federal, state and municipal level. According to the Ministry of Health (BRASIL, 2004), the maternal mortality ratio in the country in 2004 was 76.1 per 100,000 live births. The Northeast region had the highest rate, with 60.8, followed by the Centre-West region with 60.3, then the South region with 56.6, the North region with 53.2 and the lowest rate was found in the Southeast region with 45.9 (IBGE, 2008).

In the municipality of Londrina, where the study was carried out, the maternal mortality ratio in 2004 was 14, a rate well below that estimated for Brazil (76.1) for the same year. In the following years, there was a rise to 57.1 in 2005, a fall in the following two years, 14.4 in 2006 and 15.1 in 2007, and a rise again in 2008, with a significant rate of 60.46 (PARANÁ, GOVERNMENT OF THE STATE OF PARANÁ, 2008).

Despite the high numbers of maternal deaths in different regions, it is known that the coverage of the maternal mortality information system does not cover all cases, which means that maternal deaths are underreported (WHO, 2003).

It is estimated that the coverage of the maternal mortality information system is 85 per cent. However, it is known that there is underreporting and that the declaration of a maternal cause as cause of death is not entirely accurate (LAURENTI; JORGE; GOTLIEB, 2004).

Gomes, Mamede and Costa-Júnior (2004), studying the registration of maternal deaths in the states of São Paulo, Paraná, Pará, Ceará and Mato Grosso in 1999 and 2000, using the Hospital Information System of the Unified Health System (SIH-SUS), found that the system registered 596 maternal deaths during this period. However, the researchers identified another 55 cases of deaths of women of reproductive age, which should have been counted as maternal deaths, thus totalling 651 maternal deaths in that period in the states studied and not 596 as officialised. They conclude that those 55 cases were therefore unrecorded or masked maternal deaths. These findings reveal that official data is still fragile in our country.

In 2002, a study was carried out in 25 Brazilian state capitals and the Federal District, in which the estimated maternal mortality ratio found in all the capitals was 54.3 per hundred thousand live births. The study found that 67.1 per cent of deaths were due to direct obstetric causes. Hypertensive disorders predominated among the causes with 24.9 per cent. Complications of labour and delivery accounted for 10.4% of maternal deaths. Haemorrhagic complications, mainly due to placenta previa and placental abruption, accounted for 9.0% of all deaths. The researchers also identified 95 deaths of women aged 10 to 49 who had not been declared as maternal deaths in addition to the 144 official declarations (LAURENTI; JORGE; GOTLIEB, 2004).

Therefore, the real magnitude of maternal mortality in our country is not fully represented in the official figures, just like developing countries, which also have difficulties identifying these figures; even developed countries report problems, albeit to a lesser degree, in capturing all maternal deaths (WHO, 2003).

The main causes of maternal deaths are well known and more than 80 per cent of them could be prevented or could be avoided by effective and available actions, even in the world's poorest countries. This tragedy is even greater when we realise that women die during the normal period of the reproductive process and that many of these deaths could be avoided through basic preventive measures, such as identifying complications early, taking action in emergencies and using qualified personnel during the process of pregnancy, labour, birth and the puerperium (WHO, 1999; MACDONALD, STARRS, 2003).

In 1987, the Global Initiative for Risk-Free Motherhood (IMSR) was launched in response to this public health problem, led by the Inter-Agency Group for Risk-Free Motherhood, with the aim of raising awareness and promoting action at a global and national level to make pregnancies and births safer for women and their children (MACDONALD, STARRS, 2003).

In 1997, the Inter-Agency Group (IAG) convened an international conference with the aim of examining the lessons learned during the first ten years of the initiative, identifying the most effective strategies and mobilising action at national level to implement these strategies. Soon, "a clear consensus emerged on the value of skilled care during childbirth as a key intervention to make pregnancies and births safer." (MACDONALD, STARRS, 2003).

More recently, the United Nations system and its components ratified the Millennium Development Goals, which include the reduction of mortality among one of its 8 goals, with the proportion of births attended by qualified personnel. Although progress has been made in implementing the goals, there is still much to be done, which will require commitments and support from various partners, including governments, NGOs, international aid organisations and donor bodies, among others (MACDONALD, STARRS, 2003).

The education of qualified professionals and the place where they practice are essential for obtaining effective training for qualified care (MACLEAN, 2003).

With the aim of improving the quality of care for women during pregnancy and childbirth, the International Confederation of Midwives drew up the Core Competences in Midwifery. This document has been ratified by the World Health Organisation and the International Federation of Gynaecology and Obstetrics, validating it internationally.

The essential competences that a qualified professional must possess, as recommended by the International Confederation of Midwives, are:

a) <u>Competence 1</u>: midwives have the knowledge and skills required from the social sciences, public health and ethics, which form the basis of high-quality, culturally relevant, appropriate care for women, newborns and families in the reproductive period.

b) <u>Competence 2</u>: midwives provide high quality, culturally sensitive health education and services for the whole community to promote healthy family life, planned pregnancies and positive motherhood and fatherhood.

c) <u>Competence 3</u>: midwives provide high-quality antenatal care, concerned with optimising women's health during pregnancy; this includes early detection, treatment or referral of certain complications.

d) <u>Competence 4</u>: Midwives provide high-quality, culturally sensitive care during childbirth. They conduct hygienic and safe childbirth and manage emergency situations to optimise the health of women and newborns.

e) <u>Competence 5</u>: midwives offer women comprehensive, high-quality, culturally sensitive care during the postpartum period.

f) <u>Competence 6</u>: midwives provide high-quality comprehensive care for the healthy newborn, from birth to two months of age (INTERNATIONAL CONFEDERATION OF MIDWIVES, 2002).

Competences refer to personal characteristics and are defined in a context involving knowledge, acquired and inherited characteristics and skills (KAK et al, 2001). The values attributed reflect on society, on a particular career and provide guidance on the training process and professional assessment (LIMA, 2005).

It is estimated that currently only 53 per cent of women in developing countries give birth while being cared for by qualified personnel and approximately 15 per cent of pregnant women experience some life-threatening complication during pregnancy and childbirth. Health professionals must have the necessary skills to save the lives of these women with serious complications (WHO, 2003).

In order to improve the situation, the IAG Group has drawn up a multi-step strategy, centred primarily on the process of skilled care during childbirth, rather than focusing solely on staff or individual skilled providers, as a way of ensuring that the wider facilitating context in which health professionals provide maternal care is also taken into account (MACDONALD, STARRS, 2003).

Having realised this reality, international organisations have spared no effort in discussing action strategies to reverse the situation. These actions include a strong consensus that has emerged on the value of qualified care during childbirth as a fundamental intervention to make pregnancies and births safer.

In a survey carried out by region, it was identified that the percentage of births attended by a qualified person is 99 per cent in North America, 98 per cent in Europe, 75 per cent in Latin America and the Caribbean, 53 per cent in Asia, 52 per cent in Oceania and 42 per cent in Africa (WHO, 1996).

Various international and national bodies have set targets for reducing maternal mortality and expanding qualified care during childbirth. Historical experience and evidence (Sweden and the Netherlands), as well as contemporary evidence (Chile and Sri Lanka), has indicated that the development of obstetric care coverage in each country is the most important measure for reducing maternal and perinatal mortality (PAHO, 2004).

In Brazil, one of the mechanisms adopted by the government to alleviate the situation is the Ministry of Health's programme called "National Pact for the Reduction of Maternal and Neonatal Mortality", launched in March 2004, which consists of implementing a set of actions articulated by the different spheres of government for the qualification of obstetric and neonatal care, so that by the end of 2006 the current mortality rates will have been reduced by 15%. According to Dr Maria José de Araújo, coordinator of the Ministry of Health's Women's Health Department (PAHO, 2004a), "For every 100,000 live births, around 74 women die from complications during pregnancy, childbirth or the puerperium. Among the causes of these deaths are factors such as hypertension, haemorrhages, infections and abortion.

The programme's priority actions include training and continuing education for all professionals involved in obstetric and neonatal care. "The most alarming situation in Brazil today is not access to services, but the precarious quality of care," observes Dr Maria José de Araújo (PAHO, 2004b). She also adds that she hopes to increase the number of State Maternal Death Committees by 100 per cent as a strategy to solve the problem of inaccurate reporting of mortality among women during the reproductive period.

The representative of the World Health Organisation's Maternal Health programme, Enrique Ezcurra (PAHO, 2004c), says that the National Pact for the Reduction of Mortality was right to include Brazilian society in all the stages of its development. The plan was launched by the federal government in March 2004 and provides for financial support and investment in training professionals. He adds that in order to change the situation, the issue needs to be made a political priority.

Ezcurra cites Brazil and Cuba as examples. While Brazil has 74 female deaths per 100,000 live births, Cuba has 24. "For 30 years, Cuba has been taking measures, prioritising health, and is an outstanding example. The labour force in the area is qualified and at least 99% of births are carried out by specialists," he explains. According to him, the lack of qualified care is one of the main causes of death. Ezcurra says that Africa concentrates 90% of the world's deaths because it is a continent with "little economic development, few qualified medical personnel and infrastructure problems" (PAHO, 2004c).

With regard to the demand for technical and auxiliary level training in specific health functions, it is estimated that around 225,000 workers perform functions for which they are not prepared, working in nursing care in the hospital and outpatient networks. Given this situation, the Ministry of Health is developing a broad funding and technical cooperation project aimed at reducing the national deficit of qualified auxiliary nursing staff, reducing the risk of inappropriate practices and regularising the employment of staff (PAHO, 2004 d).

Mirta Roses, director of the Pan American Health Organisation (PAHO, 2004e), says that solving public health problems in the 21st century depends on addressing three objectives simultaneously. One is to resolve the unfinished agenda: "[...] these are the problems that we know how to solve, such as infant mortality, but lack resources." The other two objectives are to protect achievements - such as preventing the recurrence of controlled diseases like measles - and to tackle new challenges. He adds that in Latin America and the Caribbean, 230 million inhabitants (46 per cent) do not have health insurance, 125 million (27 per cent) lack permanent access to basic health services, 17 per cent of births do not have qualified assistance", revealing that the lack of qualification in assistance also extends to other health sectors.

According to Witt (2005), the main recommendation for reducing maternal and neonatal morbidity and mortality is that all women should be cared for by qualified staff. The importance of nursing work in primary care, expressed in the recognition that nurses have a fundamental role to play in the performance of essential public health functions, has been recognised in Brazil by managers and the population; the doubt remains with the nurses.

MacDonalds and Starrs (2003) state that historical and epidemiological evidence suggests that skilled care during childbirth and immediately afterwards can have a significant effect on reducing maternal deaths. The author adds that skilled care refers to the process by which a pregnant woman and her baby receive appropriate care during pregnancy, labour, childbirth and the postnatal and neonatal period, regardless of whether the birth takes place at home, in a health centre or in hospital. For this to happen, the provider must have the necessary skills, as well as the support of a facilitating context at various levels of the health system. This includes a framework of policies and norms, medicines and materials, adequate equipment and infrastructure, as well as an efficient and effective communication, referral and transport system. Skilled care includes care for women who suffer life-threatening complications, but is not limited to this; it can prevent some complications, increase the likelihood of prompt and appropriate treatment when complications occur, and can promote rapid and timely referral when necessary.

Based on the Joint WHO/UNFPA/UNICEF/World Bank Declaration on Reducing Maternal Mortality in Geneva in 2003, the term "skilled personnel or provider" refers exclusively to those people with expertise in professional birth care (e.g. doctors, professional midwives, nurses) who have been trained to achieve expertise in the skills needed to provide competent care during pregnancy and childbirth. Qualified people should be able to manage labour and normal birth, recognise the onset of complications, carry out essential interventions, initiate treatment and supervise the referral of mother and baby to interventions that are beyond their competence or not possible in that particular context (MACDONALD; STARRS, 2003).

However, it adds that in order to provide effective, good quality care during pregnancy and childbirth, qualified staff must have a variety of specific skills and be able to exercise them competently. It is also essential that qualified staff are authorised to carry out all the procedures for which they have been trained, in order to keep their skills up to date and offer care that meets the needs of the women for whom the services are provided. For this to happen, qualified personnel need a facilitating context in which to provide the service. This includes a supportive legal and regulatory framework, access to essential equipment and medicines, a functioning referral system and education and health systems that foster critical thinking, clinical competence and the development of effective interpersonal and communication skills (MACDONALD; STARRS, 2003).

The facilitating context referred to by the author needs to be made up of fundamental factors such as:

a) supportive policies, laws and regulations that prioritise risk-free motherhood, authorise health professionals, including traditional midwives, to carry out all those life-saving interventions in which they have competence, and counter the barriers to access to services that women face;

b) effective health system infrastructure, including adequate equipment and supplies and referral, communication and transport systems;

c) professional associations that promote the training of qualified personnel, formulate policies and protocols, establish standards of practice and basic competences, and facilitate communication and the exchange of information;

d) quality education and supervision system that offers opportunities for pre-service training and continuing education and provides a mechanism for supervision and support (MACDONALD; STARRS, 2003).

The World Health Organisation (WHO) defines a qualified birthing professional as a professional midwife (an undergraduate with specific training in obstetric care), a nurse specialising in obstetrics, or a doctor with specific expertise and experience (STARRS, 1998).

Brazil has actively participated in the Safe Motherhood Initiative, adopting a set of mechanisms to adhere to the proposal and reduce maternal and neonatal mortality at a national level.

One of the strategies proposed was the creation of the Safe Motherhood Project in 1996, a partnership between the Ministry of Health, the Brazilian Federation of Gynaecology and Obstetrics (FEBRASGO), the Pan American Health Organisation (PAHO/WHO) and UNFPA. This project, made up of eight steps to achieve safe motherhood, is an attempt to mobilise professionals who work directly or indirectly in women's care, reproductive health, as well as childcare, in order to achieve effective care and reduce maternal and infant morbidity and mortality (FEBRASGO, 1995).

With the aim of improving the quality of care provided by health professionals to women in the pregnancy-puerperium cycle, the government, through the Ministry of Health, began to offer courses to train nurses with a specialisation in obstetric nursing, enabling them to be legally able to assist women from pregnancy to normal childbirth without dystocia (BRASIL, 1986). It is known that these trained professionals are scarce in most hospitals and that labour and delivery is often assisted by generalist nurses, legal midwives or even onlookers, especially in the interior of Brazil.

The World Health Organisation considers that, due to the less interventionist characteristics of their care, professional nurses are the most suitable professionals to care for women during pregnancy and childbirth. It believes that they are the least expensive and most effective professionals for achieving safe motherhood, reducing morbidity and mortality and the costs of caring for women in the pregnancy and childbirth cycle. The Brazilian government has endeavoured to encourage the training of human resources, including obstetric nurses, in order to reverse the situation in the country through the qualification of the staff who care for women. Thus, the Ministry of Health's publication of Ordinance No. 2.815/98 reinforced the role of this professional in obstetric care at the time of childbirth, deciding to include deliveries carried out by obstetric nurses in the Unified Health System (SUS) payment table (SHIRMER, 2004).

As the number of obstetric nurses was low in our country, the Ministry of Health, in partnership with the Nursing Schools, started a movement to train nurses to carry out normal childbirth through specialisation courses in obstetric nursing in all regions of Brazil. This partnership began in 1999 and continues in 2006; more than 77 courses have already been organised across the country (SHIRMER, 2004).

Measures that are being taken to improve labour and birth care are related to encouraging and supporting the creation of normal birth centres throughout the country, investing in the qualification of maternity hospitals that carry out births and emergency services for women and newborns, as well as prioritising the training and continuing education of all professionals involved in obstetric care (SHIRMER, 2004).

During my experience on the obstetric nursing residency course and working as an obstetric nurse living with the reality of various maternity hospitals in the interior of Paraná, I realised how the nursing team acts in different ways in relation to caring for parturients, especially when comparing maternity hospitals affiliated to the Unified Health System and Supplementary Medicine.

The lack of quality in health services has been the target of criticism, as it reflects a lack of humanisation in care and high maternal and neonatal morbidity and mortality rates (MELLEIRO et al. 1998).

The difference between healthcare models has a negative impact on women's health. Our country still has a very high maternal mortality rate; there are a high number of unwanted pregnancies due to failures in family planning and caesarean section rates are gradually increasing.

The high rate of surgical deliveries is another aggravating factor in the pregnancy-puerperium process. The World Health Organisation (WHO) considers caesarean sections to be an acceptable rate of around 15%. In Brazil, it is estimated that the rates are similar to those found in Latin American countries, which is 35 per cent (VILLAR et al. 2006). In the state of Paraná, in 2005, the incidence of caesarean sections was 50.2 per cent of all deliveries, much higher than the rate stipulated by the WHO. In the same year, in the municipality of Londrina, the caesarean section rate was 56.6% (PARANÁ, GOVERNMENT OF THE STATE OF PARANÁ, 2008).

The country abuses surgical deliveries, even though it knows that this is the option in the most serious cases. There are also inaccuracies in the reporting system presented to the Unified Health System (SUS) regarding the excess of caesarean sections by health services. The International Confederation of Midwives (ICM) and the Brazilian Federation of Gynaecology and Obstetrics (FIGO) have set some targets for reducing maternal morbidity and mortality; they have proposed a target of one person for every 5,000 inhabitants who is skilled in professional childbirth care, assuming only obstetric care. In developing countries, this would mean one qualified person providing care for 200 births a year (MACDONALD; STARRS, 2003).

In this context, where maternal deaths and high rates of caesarean sections continue to be a problem to be tackled, qualified childbirth care is a fundamental strategy for making pregnancies and births safer and can make a significant contribution to reducing maternal deaths. Considering that health professionals who attend to pregnancy, labour and birth and post-natal care must have essential competences (knowledge and skills) to carry out obstetric practice with quality, we defined the competences developed by nursing staff (obstetric nurses, nurses, nursing technicians and assistants) in the care of women in the pregnancy-puerperal cycle in the city of Londrina as the object of this study.

1.3 Justification and relevance

In order to draw up a profile of obstetric care services in the selected municipality, it will be necessary to explore the extent of these services and the practices set up there. This information is necessary so that the region can assess maternal and child health services and their results in terms of the prevalence of the maternal and neonatal health care system and the model or models that shape this care.

The purpose of this research is to help identify the obstetric care models of the services that care for women in the pregnancy-puerperal cycle in the city of Londrina, state of Paraná, and in particular to verify the competences and skills developed by the nursing staff (obstetricians/obstetric nurses and others) in these services.

The International Confederation of Midwives (ICM) includes in its set of essential competences for the basic practice of midwifery the knowledge and skills that qualified professionals must have in order to provide women with qualified care at all stages of the reproductive cycle. The results of this study could help answer the following questions: Who are the nursing professionals who provide care to women during labour, childbirth and the immediate postpartum period in the municipality of Londrina? What are the actions/interventions that each nursing professional in this municipality performs in caring for mother and child during labour, childbirth and the immediate postpartum period? Are the actions carried out by nursing professionals in the municipality of Londrina based on scientific evidence? And more specifically: Is the performance of the essential competences for quality care in obstetrics in the municipality of Londrina part of the practice of nursing professionals?

Therefore, analysing the skills performed by nursing staff in caring for women in the pregnancy-puerperium cycle in the region studied will contribute to national policies for training and qualifying staff to care for women and their families during pregnancy, childbirth and postpartum, and consequently to reducing maternal and neonatal mortality.

CHAPTER 2

OBJECTIVES

2.1 General Objective

To understand the reality of nursing professionals' care for women during labour, childbirth and the immediate postpartum period in the city of Londrina.

2.2 Specific objectives

a) To characterise the nursing professionals who provide care to women during labour, childbirth and postpartum in the selected municipality.

b) To describe the profile of nursing professionals involved in caring for women during labour, childbirth and the immediate postpartum period in the selected municipality.

c) To identify the skills/actions carried out by nursing professionals in caring for women during labour, childbirth and the immediate postpartum period in the selected municipality.

CHAPTER 3

METHODOLOGY

3.1 Study characteristics

In order to find answers to these objectives, a descriptive and exploratory study was carried out, using a quantitative approach.

According to studies by Pereira (2003), descriptive epidemiological investigations aim to provide information on the distribution of an event in the population in quantitative terms. They can be incidence or prevalence studies. There is no control group for comparing the results, at least as is done in analytical studies - which is why they are considered non-controlling studies. The researcher interested in profiling a particular topic simply has to observe how these situations are occurring, in one or more populations, and express the respective frequencies appropriately.

Furthermore, in this type of study, health information can refer to the whole population or specifically to subgroups of that population.

Polit et al (2004) state that "[...] the purpose of a descriptive study is to observe, describe and document aspects of a situation." For Trivinos (1987), the intention of getting to know a certain reality is the essential focus of the descriptive study, accurately describing the facts and phenomena of that reality.

The descriptive study follows the same lines of reasoning as a scientific paper and its preparation also has a similar arrangement of themes: "introduction", "methodology", "results" and "discussion", alongside the "summary" and "bibliographical references", although these are not necessarily explicitly placed (PEREIRA, 2003).

Quantitative studies work at the level of reality, where data is presented to the senses, with the aim of providing observable indicators and trends. The exploratory study aims to fully describe a given phenomenon (MINAYO; SANCHES, 1993).

Pereira (2003) states in his studies that the proper organisation of a database makes it easier to carry out descriptive studies and that the core of this type of study is the correct determination of frequencies. He states that the better the database in terms of population coverage and the quality of its content, the more accurate the descriptive tables will be.

He adds that the results of descriptive studies are presented in tables, graphs or other forms of frequency distribution of a given event and are used to achieve two main objectives: 1) to identify risk groups, which informs about the needs and characteristics of the segments that could benefit from some form of sanitation measure; 2) to suggest explanations for variations in frequency, which serves as a basis for research on the subject, through analytical studies.

In our study, data collection was carried out through structured interviews and direct, non-participatory observation of the practice of nursing professionals, guided by previously prepared instruments based on the essential competences in midwifery (INTERNATIONAL CONFEDERATION OF MIDWIVES, 2002).

Pereira (2004) states that in order for the survey to be carried out successfully, it is necessary to have a suitable form for collecting data, so that the objectives of the investigation can be achieved.

Richardson et al. (1999) explain that in observation, the researcher only acts as a spectator, paying attention to events that are pertinent to what is being investigated. Based on the research objectives, and using an observation script, the researcher tries to see and record as many occurrences as possible that are of interest to their work.

3.2 Study site

The study was carried out in the city of Londrina. The city got its name because on 21 August 1929 the first expedition of the Companhia de

Terras Norte do Paraná to the place called Património Três Bocas, where engineer Dr Alexandre Razgulaeff set the first landmark on the land where Londrina would emerge. The city was named after London - "little London" - by Dr João Domingues Sampaio, one of the first directors of Companhia de Terras Norte do Paraná. The town was created five years later by State Decree No. 2,519, signed by Interventor Manoel Ribas on 3 December 1934. It was installed on 10 December of the same year, the date on which the town's anniversary is celebrated.

The city of Londrina is located in the interior of the state of Paraná, approximately 330 kilometres from Curitiba, the state capital. It has an estimated population of 510,707 inhabitants, with approximately 177,000 women of reproductive age (IBGE, 2008).

Londrina has grown rapidly and continuously, becoming not only a regional centre but also the third largest city in the south of the country, after Curitiba and Porto Alegre.

The city also has several Research Centres and Higher Education Institutions, including the Brazilian Agricultural Research Corporation (Embrapa), Londrina State University (UEL), Pitágoras College in Londrina, North University of Paraná (Unopar) and Philadelphia University (Unifil).

It is the first Brazilian city to have a Special Secretariat for Women, which offers social, legal and psychological assistance to women who are victims of prejudice, violence and discrimination (LONDRINA, 2007).

The city has 56 Basic Health Units, 13 of which are in rural areas and the others in urban areas, and 21 hospitals offering 1,653 beds (LONDRINA, 2007).

The municipality has five hospitals that provide care for women during labour and birth. Two of these institutions provide strictly private services, two provide services strictly through the Unified Health System (SUS) and one provides philanthropic services. In total, approximately 7,000 births are carried out every year, with a monthly average of 600 deliveries, 43% of which are vaginal and 57% caesarean sections (PARANÁ, GOVERNMENT OF THE STATE OF PARANÁ, 2007).

To collect data for this study, we selected hospital institutions with maternity services located in the city of Londrina. Three hospitals gave their consent: a public maternity hospital ("luz" maternity hospital), a public hospital ("sol" maternity hospital) and a philanthropic hospital ("lua" maternity hospital), with authorisation from their Clinical Directors. The municipality's private hospitals did not consent to the research.

3.1.1 Maternity "light

This institution is maintained by the Municipal Health Service Autarchy (ASMS), which provides services via the Unified Health System (SUS).

It was inaugurated in 1992 and attends around 75 per cent of SUS deliveries in the municipality. It is a reference point for low- and medium-risk pregnant women who have or have not had prenatal care in the basic health network.

It employs 26 doctors, including ten obstetricians, eight anaesthetists and eight paediatricians, 13 nurses and 64 nursing assistants or technicians. The nursing team works a 30-hour week. Some professionals work extra shifts to cover time off, which vary each month.

It has a multidisciplinary team made up of nurses, obstetric nurses, nursing technicians and assistants, obstetricians, paediatricians, anaesthesiologists, nutritionists and support staff.

Adhering to the system of Joint Accommodation and the non-use of artificial nipples since its implementation, the Maternity Hospital "luz" uses the promotion, protection and maintenance of Breastfeeding, having won the title of "Baby Friendly Hospital Initiative", recommended by UNICEF/WHO, on 4th July 2000.

In 2006, the Maternity received the Galba de Araújo award from the Ministry of Health to highlight hospitals that invest the most in normal childbirth and humanised care for pregnant women and babies.

In 2008, 3,622 births were carried out, of which 2,662 were normal births and 957 were caesarean sections, showing a caesarean section rate of 25.5 per cent.

Its physical structure includes a reception, a pre-natal and delivery unit, an obstetric centre, a material centre, a newborn unit, a rooming-in unit and an administrative area.

The antepartum and labour unit consists of two rooms for admission consultations, where the doctor or medical student provides care. The presence of a carer is permitted at this time. The nursing team participates by carrying out the initial approach and checking for HOS, collecting tests when necessary. This ward is divided by a door and the next room houses the antepartum and labour rooms. Cardiotocography (CTG) is carried out in all the rooms; there are two specific areas equipped with comfortable armchairs. The nurse installs the equipment and removes it after the specified time. Companions are not allowed. After the test, the pregnant woman returns to the ward and waits for the doctor to finish.

After the assessment, when the need for hospitalisation is detected, the pregnant woman is referred to the antepartum ward by the nursing assistant or technician. The Hospital Admission Authorisation (AIH) is generated in the name of the doctor on duty.

There are 8 beds in the antepartum ward, divided into three rooms. The first room holds four patients; it is equipped with a bathroom for the exclusive use of the pregnant women admitted (toilet, sink and shower). The beds are separated by fixed screens and there is a mobile screen, all illustrated with information on humanisation practices and the development of childbirth. In this room there is also a U-shaped stool, a horse and two balls for doing exercises and helping with labour. The second and third rooms are similar, with only two beds in each.

Analgesia for normal childbirth is not performed very often, as there is only one anaesthetist on duty.

In the same environment, there are three delivery rooms, one of which is equipped with a differentiated table that allows the parturient greater freedom to change position. This room is mostly used for deliveries assisted by obstetric nurses. The composition of the rooms is practically the same: gynaecological table, heated cot, neonatal resuscitation material, adult stethoscope and sphygmomanometer, medicines and surgical materials, oxygen network, suction and piped compressed air.

After the birth, the newborn is taken to the hygiene room, where they receive initial care and their first bath. The puerperal woman awaits the end of labour in the delivery room and, after being released by the team that assisted her, remains on a stretcher in the corridor, watching the procedures carried out on her child. After the newborn has been cared for, the couple waits to be released by the antepartum nurse; they then request a place in the rooming-in unit. The rooming-in nurse releases a team of staff to collect and house the couple.

If the newborn needs to be observed, there is an inpatient unit with five beds and equipped with an infant respirator, incubators and a heated cot. When the newborn's general condition is more serious, they are transferred to an Intensive Care Unit in another, larger hospital.

The shared accommodation consists of 36 beds organised as follows: in two rooms there is capacity for three binomials, in the others there is capacity for two. The rooms are equipped with armchairs and a bathroom.

Newborns are vaccinated against hepatitis B and BCG. They are given the heel prick test and before they are discharged they have their birth certificate made, as there is an agreement with the city's registry offices to do this.

There is also the Rosa Viva programme, which treats female victims of sexual violence from the age of 12. The nurse and doctor on duty provide emergency care in the first 72 hours, collect secretions and tests and make the appropriate referrals to the police station, psychological care and the forensic medical institute, if necessary.

3.1.2   Maternity sunshine

The institution was created in 1970 to meet the needs of the State University of Londrina's medical course, which required a teaching hospital. It is a reference hospital for Londrina and the region for high-calibre care.

It is considered the third largest teaching hospital in southern Brazil. It currently has a capacity of 311 beds, distributed among various medical specialities, totally at the disposal of the Unified Health System.

Its facilities include a Haemocentre and a Human Milk Bank.

The Hospital das Clínicas Outpatient Clinic (AHC) is part of its organisational structure and sees an average of 7,300 patients per month. It also provides high-risk prenatal care, where it is a reference for pregnant women coming from the primary healthcare network in Londrina and the region.

In 2000, it received the Child-Friendly Hospital Initiative award and in the same year the Hospital Management and Care Quality award, all given by the Ministry of Health for excellent services rendered.

In 2008, 889 deliveries were carried out at the hospital, of which 603 were caesarean sections and the rest (286) were normal deliveries. The caesarean section rate is close to 68 per cent and is justified by the care of high-risk patients.

Pregnant women are first seen in the obstetric emergency department (on the ground floor) and, if there is a need for hospitalisation, they are referred to the maternity ward, which is on the upper floor. The nurse in charge of this sector supervises two other wards.

The maternity ward has 19 beds, divided into two rooms with six beds each, one room with three beds and two rooms with two beds. There are only two bathrooms in this ward.

Parturients are seen by the medical team and all obstetric checks are carried out by them.

There is a newborn care room equipped with a heated cot and equipment for initial care (bathing, measurements, vitamin K application) and oxygen application when necessary.

There is a delivery room equipped with two gynaecological tables in the same room, so that two births can take place simultaneously; there is no partition with screens. Most of the time, escorts are not allowed. Inside the delivery room, away from the parturient's view, there is a room where the newborn is welcomed.

If the birth is normal, the puerperal woman is then sent to the rooming-in unit and breastfeeding begins. As the maternity hospital is a referral centre for high-risk pregnant women, many deliveries are operative. In the case of a caesarean section, the puerperal woman returns to the ward after recovering from the anaesthetic; in this case, the newborn stays in the support room in the maternity ward.

The nurses work a 36-hour shift and at the weekend and at night they provide care in the Neonatal Intensive Care Unit and the Intermediate Care Unit. These sectors are in another wing of the hospital.

3.1.3 Maternity moon

It is a philanthropic hospital with an emphasis on high-risk pregnant women. It has 217 beds, 124 of which are allocated to SUS.

The institution has 32 maternity beds, 6 of which are for SUS services, a reception room, an inpatient ward, an intermediate and intensive care unit for newborns and two delivery rooms. When operative deliveries are necessary, they take place in the surgical centre in another wing of the hospital.

In 2008, 1,311 births were carried out at this institution, of which 1,125 were caesarean sections and 186 normal, showing a caesarean section rate of 85.8 per cent in this period.

Pregnant women with a SUS contract only receive care if they are referred by a support service, SAMU (Mobile Emergency Care Service), SIATE (Integrated Emergency Trauma Care System), or if they have been transferred from another institution. Direct referral is permitted if the pregnant woman has another health insurance plan or presents private care.

The nurse is the professional who provides the first care for the pregnant woman. Sometimes the doctor sends a request for hospitalisation and obstetric care is not provided in the assessment room. The nurse carries out the general and obstetric physical examination, performs the cardiotocography, performs the vaginal examination and informs the doctor. The on-call SUS doctor stays at a distance and turns up for assessments when there is a demand.

The hospitalisation is determined by the doctor, who requests the Authorisation for Hospital Admission.

There are two separate delivery rooms in the sector, equipped with a gynaecological table and equipment for caring for the newborn. The nurse only delivers babies in the doctor's absence.

After the birth, the newborn is taken to a support room, where initial procedures such as bathing, measurements, vitamin K application and nursing notes are carried out. This room is equipped with oxygen, an aspirator and piped compressed air. There are also incubators and heated cots.

If the labour is normal, the patient is taken to the operating theatre afterwards. In the case of a caesarean section, the puerperal woman remains in the operating theatre for an average of three hours.

The nursing team works a 42-hour week. The night nurse also takes charge of the paediatric ward and the newborn unit.

3.3 Ethical Aspects of Research

This study complied with the requirements of Resolution 196/96 of the National Health Council on research involving human beings. It was approved by the Research Ethics Committee (CEP) of the Ribeirão Preto Nursing School of the University of São Paulo (EERP - USP) under protocol no. 265/2008 (Annex 1).

A "Free and Informed Consent Form" was drawn up with information about the research, in simple and objective language, for the professionals studied and the participating institutions, also covering the purposes of the research, the procedures and benefits, the guarantee of anonymity, respect for the desire to participate in the study, giving them the freedom to stop participating in the research as soon as they wish, without this causing personal and/or professional harm to themselves or the institution to which they are linked.

A "Free and Informed Consent Form" was also drawn up for the parturients, asking for their consent to observe their labour and delivery. The form contains information about the research, in simple and objective language, and guarantees anonymity; the possibility of not allowing observation at any time was made clear.

It was also made clear that the data obtained would be used for scientific research, for statistical purposes, and possible publication at a later date.

After explaining the "Informed Consent Form", those who agreed were asked to sign it.

3.4 Research Subjects

Nursing professionals (obstetric nurses, nurses, nursing technicians and assistants) working in women's health care services during labour and delivery in the selected hospitals took part in this study.

3.5 Data Collection

In order to analyse the maternal and child health situation in Londrina, a survey was carried out in the administrative sectors of the institutions on the number of beds, the number of procedures carried out, the number of professionals working in childbirth care and their training, and the operating rules of the institutions.

Data was collected between January and March 2009 at the three participating health centres.

Data collection took place in two stages:

In the first stage, we characterised the nursing professionals who provide care to women during labour, childbirth and the immediate postpartum period through structured interviews with the subjects of this study (nursing assistants, nursing technicians, nurses and nurses specialising in obstetrics), with the aim of obtaining socio-demographic information and identifying the functions and activities carried out by these professionals.

To collect data for this stage of the study, an "Instrument for interviewing nursing professionals" (Appendix II) was used, with a script aimed at collecting specific information about their professional profile, consisting of open and closed questions, adapted from Dotto's work (2006).

The participants were interviewed only after being informed of the study's objectives and signing the "Informed Consent Form for Nursing Professionals" (Appendix III). The interview took place in the professional's workplace, in direct contact with the researcher, and lasted an average of 15 minutes.

At this stage, professionals who were absent due to holidays or leave on the days intended for data collection were excluded.

The second stage of data collection involved non-participatory and structured observation of the care provided to parturient and puerperal women: identifying the actions carried out by nursing professionals in the care of parturient women, through non-participatory and structured direct observation of the context of this care. A previously prepared observation script was used: the "Observation script: antepartum, labour and puerperium" (Appendix IV). This instrument, designed specifically for this purpose, had already been tested and used by Dotto (2006) and was structured in the form of a checklist. The nursing professionals taking part in this stage were included in the research only after signing the "Informed Consent Form for Nursing Professionals" (Appendix III). In the same way, the women being cared for were informed about the objectives of the research; after consenting, they signed the "Informed Consent Form for Parturient Women" (Appendix V) and took part in the research.

A previously trained trainee took part in this stage. The pilot test was applied as a way of improving and making the necessary corrections. The observations were carried out by the researcher and a trainee, in search of a representative sample of the reality being studied. The researcher was present during the morning shifts (from 7am to 1pm), afternoon shifts (from 1pm to 7pm), even and odd night shifts (7pm to 1am). A total of 60 shifts of 6 hours of observation each were carried out, 20 shifts in each institution.

Another established criterion was to observe the four stages of parturition (admission, labour, delivery and postpartum) on all shifts. This made it possible to observe 92 deliveries sequentially at all times. No patients under the age of 18 took part.

In deliveries attended by the medical team, only the activities carried out by the nursing team were observed, as this was the aim of this study.

3.6 Data Analysis

Microsoft Office Exceli 2007 was used to tabulate the descriptive statistics and present the data. Frequency, percentage and mean were used for the results.

The data was analysed based on the documents that underpin qualified childbirth care. These are: The Ministry of Health's Manual for Childbirth, Abortion and the Puerperium - Humanised Care for Women, the Practical Guide to Normal Childbirth Care (WHO), the Integrated Pregnancy and Birth Management (INPAC) guidelines and the core competences published by the ICM/WHO/PAHO.

CHAPTER 4

RESULTS

4.1 Characterisation of the nursing team that assists women during labour, delivery and the immediate postpartum period

The population of this study was made up of 63 nursing professionals who provide care to parturients in the maternity hospitals studied. Table 1 shows the nursing professionals involved in caring for parturients in the maternity hospitals in the city of Londrina. They are distributed as follows: 19 professionals in the "moon" maternity hospital, 20 professionals in the "sun" maternity hospital team and 24 professionals in the "light" team.

Table 1 - Distribution of nursing professionals at maternity hospitals in Londrina (PR), according to the maternity hospital surveyed.

Maternity	Nurse	Obstetric Nurse	Nursing assistant	Nursing Technician	TOTAL
"moon"	02	02	10	05	19
"sun"	03	01	06	10	20
"light"	-	05	12	07	24

Source: Londrina, 2009

This group of professionals is female (63), with an average age of 38.1 years. With regard to marital status, 43 professionals (68.3%) were married or living with a steady partner; 1 professional was widowed. Most of the professionals had financial dependents (Table 2).

Table 2 - Distribution of nursing professionals at maternity hospitals in Londrina (PR), according to age, marital status and number of children.

Variables	Category	Moon	Sun	Light	Total F	Total %
Sex	Female	19	20	24	63	100
Age	20 - 29 years	9	1	2	12	19,0
	30 - 39 years	5	10	5	20	31,8
	40 - 49 years	3	8	13	24	38,1
	50 - 60 years	2	1	4	7	11,1
Marital status	Married	9	16	12	37	58,8
	Divorced	1	2	4	7	11,1
	Single	5	-	7	12	19,0
	Consensual union	4	1	1	6	9,5
	Widow	0	1	-	1	1,6
	None	9	1	3	13	20,6

Financial dependents	1					
	2	6	7	7	20	31,8
	3	3	7	10	20	31,8
		1	5	4	10	15,8

Source: Londrina, 2009

Remuneration at the institutions surveyed ranged from R$ 1700.00 to R$ 2950.00 for nurses, from R$ 1700.00 to R$ 3235.00 for obstetric nurses and, among mid-level professionals, from R$ 650.00 to R$ 2200.00 for nursing assistants and R$ 675.00 to R$ 2300.00 for nursing technicians, as reported by the professionals and illustrated in Table 3.

When we compare the institutions surveyed, we can see that there is a big difference in salary between the professionals studied. The team of professionals at the "luz" maternity hospital who have completed high school are paid more than the team of nurses at the "lua" maternity hospital. This fact becomes clearer when we look at the average salaries by category for each of the institutions surveyed, as shown in Figure 1.

It's worth remembering that at the time of data collection, the minimum wage was R$465.00.

Table 3 - Distribution of nursing professionals at maternity hospitals in Londrina (PR), according to remuneration at the institution surveyed

REMUNERATION AT THE INSTITUTION (R$)	Nurse		Obstetric Nurse			Nursing assistant			Nursing Technician		
	Moon	Sunlight	Sun	Moon	Light	Moon	Sun	Light	Moon	Sun	Light
From 500 to 1000						10			5		
From 1001 to 1500								2			
From 1501 to 2000	2		2				4	5		7	2
From 2001 to 2500		1					2	5		3	5
From 2501 to 3000		2			4						
Above 3000				1	1						
TOTAL	2	3	2	1	5	10	6	12	5	10	7

Source: Londrina, 2009

As for the daily working hours, in the "luz" maternity hospital the professionals work 30 hours a week, in the "sol" maternity hospital the working hours are 36 hours a week and in the "lua" maternity hospital, the professionals work the longest daily hours among the maternity hospitals surveyed, 42 hours a week.

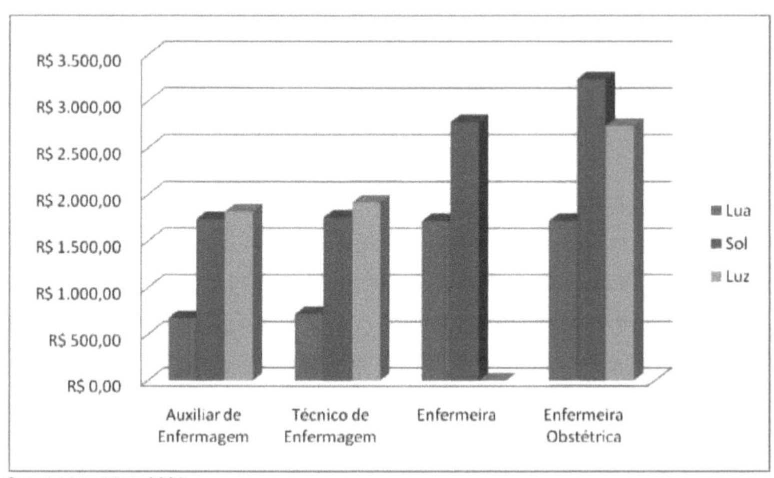

Source: Londrina, 2009

Figure 1- Average salary of nursing professionals in maternity hospitals in Londrina (PR)

When we analysed the educational level of the nursing professionals who work in childbirth care, we found five nurses who had completed a degree in nursing, but had not completed a postgraduate degree in obstetrics. The nursing technicians have completed high school, but three of them have completed a degree in nursing. Table 4 shows the length of professional training of the nursing staff at the institutions investigated.

Table 4 - Distribution of nursing professionals at maternity hospitals in Londrina (PR), according to years of training.

YEARS OF TRAINING	Nursing professionals			
	Nurse	Obstetric Nurse	Nursing assistant	Nursing Technician
Less than 1 year	-	-	-	-
1 to 2 years	-	-	12	**12**
3 to 4 years	**03**	02	10	**6**
5 to 6 years 7 to 8 years 9 to 10 years	02	05	06	4
More than 10 years	-	**01**		-
TOTAL	**05**	**08**	**28**	**22**

Source: Londrina, 2009

Of the thirteen nurses interviewed, five had specialised in obstetric nursing through funding from the Ministry of Health's Women's Thematic Area. The eight obstetric nurses who took part in the study reported having completed a specialisation in obstetric nursing with more than 360 hours. In addition to this specialisation, two nurses have specialised in Family Health and Nursing Auditing, one nurse has specialised in Neonatal Nursing and another nurse has specialised in Collective

Health, all specialisations with more than 360 hours. None of the nurses had a postgraduate degree.

The average weekly working hours of nursing professionals is 64.25 hours, ranging from 30 hours to 112 hours a week. It can be seen that in the "lua" maternity hospital, all 19 professionals work more than 40 hours a week, as can be seen in Figure 2. It was noted that 20 (32%) professionals have two or more jobs (1 nurse, 3 obstetric nurses, 8 nursing technicians and 8 nursing assistants)

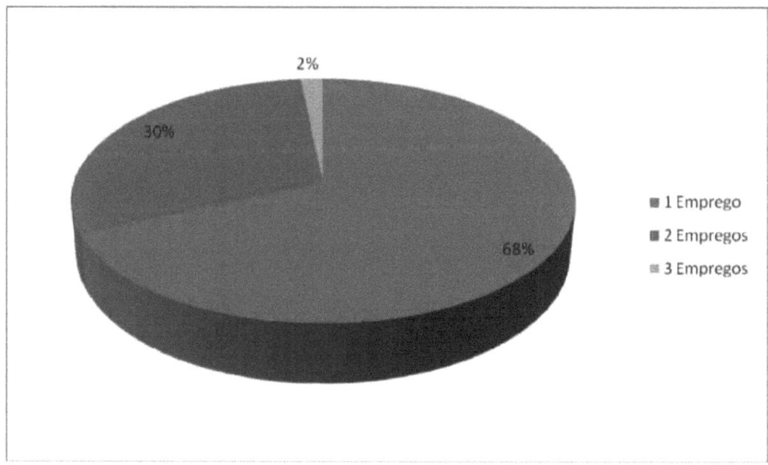

Source: Londrina, 2009

Figure 2 - Distribution of nursing professionals at maternity hospitals in Londrina (PR), according to number of jobs.

The length of professional experience in caring for women in labour and childbirth, as shown in Table 5, ranged from 7 to 265 months, with an average of 102.3 months. It can be seen that the nursing professionals who work in the "luz" maternity hospital have the longest experience in the area.

Table 5 - Distribution of nursing professionals at maternity hospitals in Londrina (PR), according to the length of time they have worked in childbirth care.

WORKING TIME	Nurse		Obstetric Nurse			Nursing assistant			Nursing Technician		
	Moon	Sunlight	Moon	Sun	Light	Moon	Sun	Light	Moon	Sun	Light
Less than 12 months	2										
12 to 24 months									2		
24 to 36 months						3			3		
36 to 48 months		1	1								
48 to 60 months		2	1			4					
60 to 72 months				1		1	4			7	
72 to 84 months							2			3	
84 to 96 months											

96 to 108 months	-	- -	-	-	1	1	-	1	-	-	-
108 to 120 months	-	- -	-	-	1	-	-	2	-	-	2
More than 120 months	-	- -	-	-	3	1	-	9	-	-	5
TOTAL	2	3	2	1	5	10	6	12	5	10	7

Source: Londrina, 2009

With regard to the commitment to updating professional practice over the last five years, Table 6 shows that the professionals who took part in the most updating events were those from the "luz" maternity hospital, with the most frequent course being Humanised Childbirth Care.

Table 6 - Distribution of nursing professionals at maternity hospitals in the city of Londrina (PR), according to refresher courses taken in the last five years.

REFRESHER COURSE	Moon	Sun	Light
Breastfeeding Day	-	02	05
Neonatal resuscitation	03	-	10
Humanised Childbirth Care	-	-	24
Latin American Obstetrics Congress	-	01	01
Brazilian Congress on Vertical Transmission	01	-	03
Breastfeeding Symposium	-	05	02
Gynaecology and Obstetrics Conference	-	02	01
Total	04	10	46

Source: Londrina, 2009

Of the 63 professionals interviewed, 40 said they had not learnt how to deliver babies. Of the 23 who had learnt, 19 said they had learnt from higher education professionals. Only three obstetric nurses reported working in childbirth, all of whom belonged to the "luz" maternity hospital. The obstetric nurses reported that they carry out normal births without dystocia, and indicate the use of oxytocin at some point during labour, according to need, usually to shorten the expulsive period, which is discussed with the doctor on duty.

With regard to the procedures carried out at the time of delivery, 100% said that they performed episiotomy when necessary, using local anaesthesia for this practice. They all reported performing episorrhaphy. Pudendal nerve block is not part of the professional practice of obstetric nurses who deliver babies in the institutions surveyed.

All the professionals who carry out births at the institution said that they do so regardless of the presence of a doctor, but all births are recorded on the hospital admission form - AIH - as a procedure carried out by a medical professional.

4.2 Characterisation of obstetric care: description of what was observed in the admission, antepartum, delivery and immediate postpartum units

During this stage, 92 deliveries were observed sequentially, during admission, during labour and delivery and in the immediate postpartum period, in all the institutions surveyed. In the "luz" maternity hospital, 60 pregnant women were observed (50 evolved to vaginal delivery and 10 to caesarean section); in the "sol" maternity hospital, 16 pregnant women were observed (10 evolved to caesarean section and 6 to vaginal delivery); and in the "lua" maternity hospital, 16 pregnant women were observed (2 evolved to vaginal delivery and 14 evolved to caesarean section).

We found that in the "luz" and "sol" maternity wards, the medical professional is responsible for admission; the team of nursing professionals only carry out the SSWs and collect tests when requested. In the "moon" maternity hospital, nursing assistants and technicians attended to the 16 births observed; the nurse did not take part in welcoming the patients, but only had contact with the patient in the postpartum period.

With regard to the presence of a companion during the birth process, we can see that in the "sun" and "moon" maternity wards there are no companions at any stage of the birth process. In the "luz" maternity hospital, the companion is allowed throughout the process, routinely in vaginal births; only in caesarean sections, the companion waits on admission and after the birth meets the patient in the support room to accompany the newborn's bath.

It was also observed that, in the three institutions surveyed, the Hospital Admission Authorisation (AIH) forms are filled in and signed by the doctor.

4.2.1 Admission of the parturient

Ninety-two admission examinations were observed during the data collection period in the morning, afternoon and even and odd night periods. In the "luz" maternity hospital, 60 admission examinations were observed, and in the "sol" and "lua" maternity hospitals, 16 admissions were observed in each institution.

Table 7 shows the frequency of activities carried out during the admission of 92 pregnant women by health professionals in the institutions studied.

Among the activities carried out, we observed that the referral of pregnant women to the examination room and the measurement of blood pressure were carried out for all pregnant women in the three institutions studied.

We found that trichotomy and enema have been abolished as routine obstetric procedures in the maternity hospitals participating in this study.

We could see that the entire admission procedure was the responsibility of the nursing assistants and technicians and the medical professional; both the nurse and the obstetric nurse were not involved in this process.

It is worth pointing out that the vaginal examination was carried out more than once on each pregnant woman in the "luz" and "sol" maternity hospitals; all the examinations were carried out by the medical team. This fact can be explained by the fact that these two institutions are training grounds for undergraduate medical students at the State University of Londrina.

Some activities were not carried out for pregnant women in any of the three institutions surveyed, such as identifying themselves to the pregnant woman and checking the woman's age. In the "lua" maternity hospital, all the admission procedures were carried out by the nursing assistants and technicians.

It is interesting to note that uterine dynamics is not a practice that is frequently carried out on admission of pregnant women by any professional category in the maternity hospitals studied, with doctors only carrying it out on 16 pregnant women in the "luz" maternity hospital. Another fact that draws attention is the low number of gestational age calculations carried out, both by amenorrhoea time and by ultrasound, as the nursing team did not carry out this practice on any of the pregnant women in the three institutions surveyed.

Table 7 - Frequency distribution of activities carried out by health professionals at maternity hospitals in Londrina (PR), according to professional category, during the admission of the 92 pregnant women observed.

Activity	Nursing assistant			Nursing Technician			Doctor or Medical Student			TOTAL
	Moon	Sun	Light	Moon	Sun	Light	Moon	Sun	Light	
The pregnant woman is identified	-	-	-	-	-	-	-	-	-	-
Refer the pregnant woman to the examination room	6	3	42	10	6	13	-	7	5	92
Apply for a pre-Christmas card	-	-	12	-	-	11	-	16	37	76
Blood pressure measurement	10	7	47	6	7	13	-	2	-	92
Question the complaint of the moment	2	-	10	3	-	12	-	16	36	79
Calculates gestational age based on amenorrhoea	-	-	-	-	-	-	-	16	60	76
Calculates gestational age based on USG	-	-	-	-	-	-	-	16	36	52
Check the age of the pregnant woman	-	-	-	-	-	-	-	-	-	-
Vaginal touch	-	-	-	-	-	-	-	24	138	162
Auscultation of BCF	10	-	-	6	-	-	-	16	52	84
Obstetric palpation	-	-	-	-	-	-	-	3	12	15
Diagnosis of labour	-	-	-	-	-	-	-	16	36	52
Uterine Dynamics	-	-	-	-	-	-	-	16	-	16
Amnioscopy	-	-	-	-	-	-	-	2	16	18
Indicates cardiotocography	-	-	-	-	-	-	-	6	53	59
Cardiotocography	-	7	40	-	7	12	-	2	-	68
TOTAL	28	17	151	25	20	61	-	158	481	941

Source: Londrina, 2009

When we analysed the total number of activities carried out in the institutions participating in this study, we found that 32.1% (302) of the total admission activities for parturient women in the maternity hospitals surveyed during the data collection period were carried out by nursing assistants and technicians.

4.2.2 Observation in labour

During the observation of pregnant women in labour, we saw that at maternity hospital "luz", 50 pregnant women progressed to normal delivery and 10 underwent caesarean section; at maternity hospital "sol", 10 progressed to caesarean section and 6 to vaginal delivery; and at maternity hospital "lua", 14 pregnant women underwent caesarean section and only 2 progressed to vaginal delivery.

Table 8 shows the frequency distribution of the activities carried out by health professionals, according to professional category, during the care of the 92 women in labour. Taking into account the total number of activities carried out (1928), we can see that the nursing team carried out around 60 per cent (1145) of the procedures.

Among the activities observed were those carried out most frequently during labour: checking the fetal heart rate (FHR) with 51.8% (1000) of the total number of procedures carried out in the three institutions, followed by vaginal touch, with 11.6% (225).

We observed that non-pharmacological pain relief procedures are not part of the routine in the "sun" and "moon" maternity wards. In the "light" maternity unit, the nursing team encourages the practice of various activities, such as relaxation baths (100), encouraging walking (42), massage (36), ball exercises (80) and horse riding (10), totalling 13.9% (268).

Table 8 - Frequency distribution of activities carried out by health professionals at maternity hospitals in Londrina (PR), according to professional category, during the pre-natal period of the 92 parturients observed.

Activity	Nursing Assistant and Technician			Nurse and Obstetrician			Doctor or Medical Student			TOTAL
	Moon	Sun	Light	Moon	Sun	Light	Moon	Sun	Light	
Take a bath	16	6	54	-	-	2	-	-	-	78
Auscultation of BCF	16	-	448	-	-	28	-	16	492	1000
Offers liquids	-	-	65	-	-	52	-	-	-	117
Offer food	-	-	12	-	-	22	-	-	-	34
Measures blood pressure	10	5	19	-	-	3	-	-	-	37
Performs vaginal touch	-	-	-	13	-	64	-	-	148	225
Checks uterine dynamics	-	-	-	2	-	12	-	-	12	26
Massage	-	-	-	-	-	36	-	-	-	36
Take a relaxing bath	-	-	52	-	-	48	-	-	-	100
Referral for ambulation	-	-	26	-	-	16	-	-	-	42
Use the ball	-	-	34	-	-	46	-	-	-	80
Use the horse	-	-	4	-	-	6	-	-	-	10
Refer for analgesia	-	-	-	-	-	-	-	-	-	-
Requests administration of oxytocin	-	-	-	-	-	-	5	6	34	45
Requests administration of other medicines	-	-	-	-	-	-	-	-	-	-
Indicates amniotomy	-	-	-	-	-	2	-	-	10	12
Use the partogram	-	-	-	-	-	26	-	-	60	86
TOTAL	42	11	714	15	-	363	5	22	756	1928

Source: Londrina, 2009

We noticed the absence of some activities for parturient women, such as measuring uterine height and abdominal circumference and performing analgesia, which are important for the quality of care provided.

Amniotomy was only indicated 12 times, all at the "luz" maternity hospital, and on two occasions the obstetric nurse indicated artificial rupture.

The use of pharmacological methods for pain relief during labour and delivery was not observed in any of the three maternity hospitals in this study.

We observed that when vaginal touch was performed (225), cervical dilation was the most frequently performed parameter (186), followed by foetal descent (45). There were no references to the characteristics of the pelvis or the variety of positions.

There were 45 indications for oxytocin, all made by doctors, 5 times in the "moon" maternity hospital, 6 times in the "sun" maternity hospital and 34 times in the "light" maternity hospital.

Uterine dynamics is a practice that is rarely used (26) to assess labour in the institutions studied in this research.

We highlight the lack of use of the partogram in the "moon" and "sun" maternity wards. In the "luz" maternity hospital, notes on the progress of labour were taken by both obstetric nurses and doctors in 100% of the deliveries observed during data collection.

It is worth noting that in practice, obstetric nurses are more active (363) in controlling labour in the "luz" maternity hospital. We also observed that the way obstetric nurses work in the "sun" and "moon" maternity wards is through bureaucratic work and little assistance.

4.2.3   Observation during vaginal delivery and immediate postpartum period

A total of 58 vaginal births were observed, of which 50 took place in the "luz" maternity hospital, six in the "sol" maternity hospital and two in the "lua" maternity hospital.

Of the births carried out during the observation period in the maternity hospitals taking part in this study, 52 were attended by doctors and six were attended by obstetric nurses. Table 9 shows the frequency distribution of births carried out by health professionals in the maternity hospitals studied.

In none of the vaginal deliveries could the parturient choose the position she wanted to give birth in; all were carried out in the lithotomy position, with the mother's back in a horizontal position, her thighs flexed and supported by leggings. The parturients were also not given any liquids. An accompanying person was present at all deliveries.

Table 9 - Distribution of the frequency of vaginal deliveries carried out by health professionals at maternity hospitals in Londrina (PR), according to professional category.

| Maternity | Health professionals | | | | | |
| | Doctor | | Obstetrician | | TOTAL | |
	n	%	n	%	n	%
"moon"	2	3,5	0	0	2	3,5
"sun"	6	10,3	0	0	6	10,3
"light"	44	75,9	6	10,3	50	86,2
TOTAL	52	89,7	6	10,3	58	100,0

Source: Londrina, 2009

Table 10 below shows the frequency of activities carried out by health professionals during the observation of the expulsion period of the 58 parturients assisted in the institutions studied.

Table 10 - Frequency distribution of activities carried out by health professionals at maternity hospitals in Londrina (PR), according to professional category, during the expulsion period of the 58 parturients observed.

Activity	Nursing Assistant and Technician			Nurse and Obstetrician			Doctor or Medical Student			TOTAL
	Moo n	Sun	Light	Sun	Moon	Light	Moon	Sun	Light	
Pull stimulus	2	2	4	-	-	12	-	-	30	50
Episiotomy	-	-	-	-	-	-	2	6	46	54
Anaesthesia before episiotomy	-	-	-	-	-	-	2	6	46	54
Use of medication: oxytocin	-	-	-	-	-	-	2	6	20	28
Kristeller manoeuvre	1	-	10	-	-	5	-	-	-	16
Perineal protection	-	-	-	-	-	6	2	6	26	40
TOTAL	3	2	14	-	-	23	8	24	168	242

Source: Londrina, 2009

The Kristeller manoeuvre was performed on 16 (27.5%) parturients, each time by the nursing team; 15 took place in the "light" maternity ward and 1 in the "moon" maternity ward.

Oxytocin was prescribed for 50 deliveries, all of which were attended by doctors. No oxytocin was prescribed for parturients assisted by obstetric nurses.

Episiotomy was performed in 93.1% (54) of the vaginal deliveries observed, but it was not performed in the deliveries attended by obstetric nurses. It is worth remembering that local anaesthesia was used before episiotomy in 100% (54) of the deliveries observed. Perineal protection was performed in 68.9% (40) of the deliveries observed during the study. In the postpartum period, we observed the fourth clinical period of labour, which takes place in the first hour after delivery, in the 58 vaginal deliveries attended during the data collection period. Table 11 shows the activities carried out during this period, according to professional category. We emphasise that the activities were carried out exclusively by the nursing team in the three institutions surveyed.

Table 11 - Frequency distribution of activities carried out by health professionals at maternity hospitals in Londrina (PR), according to professional category, during the postpartum care of the 58 puerperal women observed.

Activity	Nursing Assistant and Technician			Nurse and Obstetrician			Doctor or Medical Student			TOTAL
	Moo n	Sun	Light	Moon	Sun	Light	Moon	Sun	Light	
Obs. uterine consistency	-	-	12	-	-	-	-	-	-	12
Note: Bleeding	-	-	16	-	-	12	-	-	-	28
Uterine height	-	-	4	-	-	10	-	-	-	14
Blood pressure	-	-	26	-	-	-	-	-	-	26
TOTAL	-	-	58	-	-	22	-	-	-	80

Source: Londrina, 2009

We observed that puerperal care during the fourth clinical period is non-existent in the "sun" and "moon" maternity wards, and very little carried out in the "light" maternity ward. Among the least verified practices are the observation of uterine consistency (12) and checking uterine height. It's worth pointing out that discharge to the rooming-in ward is the responsibility of the obstetric nurse in the "luz" maternity ward, who, as we observed, is limited to checking the medical records and the documents in them.

When welcoming the newborn, we saw that in the three maternity hospitals participating in this study, the obstetric nurse, the nursing technician and the paediatrician were responsible for the care provided. Mother-child contact in the first half hour, skin-to-skin contact, suctioning the upper airways and drying the newborn were routine activities in the institutions surveyed.

CHAPTER 5

DISCUSSION

5.1 The nursing team

The nursing professionals who provide care to parturient women in the institutions studied in the city of Londrina are characterised by being exclusively female (100%); the majority are in stable marriages (68.3%), with an average age of 38.1 years. In addition, 79.4 per cent had experienced motherhood. These data are similar between the three institutions surveyed. The population studied was also characterised by a long period of professional experience and extensive weekly working hours due to the low level of pay. These data are similar to the study carried out by Dotto (2006) in the municipality of Rio Branco/AC, where the professionals who attend childbirth are people who have passed the age of 40, live with a sexual partner, have had children and have long professional experience.

With regard to working hours, 68% of nursing professionals have a job, which differs from the reality found by Fornazari (2009) in the municipality of Piracicaba/SP, where 80.7% of workers have a job. Similar data, however, was found in Rio Branco/AC by Dotto and in Araraquara/SP by Cagnin (2008), where, in both cases, 68 per cent of nursing professionals had a job.

In this study, 13 (20.6%) of the sample had higher education qualifications, 5 (7.9%) of whom were nurses and 8 (12.6%) obstetric nurses. There was a predominance of mid-level professionals, totalling 50 (79.3%). These findings are similar to the data found by Fornazari (2009), in which the percentage of professionals with higher education was 21 per cent and those with secondary education 79 per cent. However, this contrasts with the findings of Dotto (2006), in which 30% of the professionals were university graduates; Cagnin (2008), in a similar study carried out in Araraquara/SP, found that 54.5% of the nurses were specialists.

In Latin American countries, there is a predominance of mid-level professionals in the nursing workforce, with the composition varying between 52.7% and 87.8% of nursing assistants and technicians. Only Panama, Mexico and Puerto Rico differ from these figures, with a rate of less than 50% (PAN AMERICAN HEALTH ORGANISATION, PAHO, 2005).

The practice of nursing as a profession in the maternity hospitals surveyed is governed by Decree No. 94.406 of 8 June 1987, which regulates Law No. 7.498 of 25 June 1986, which provides for the practice of nursing and allows qualified professionals to practice the profession before registering with the Regional Nursing Council of the region in which they work (BRASIL, 2002).

Nursing in hospitals is characterised by long working hours and stress: night work, shift rotas, generating physical and mental overload. There is also the existence of a double working day, as they are also spouses and mothers, creating multiple roles and social demands. According to Spindola and Santos (2003), women feel overburdened by the accumulation of these roles, despite valuing their professional activities (SPINDOLA; SANTOS, 2003).

The average working hours found in this study was 64.25 hours, very similar to that found by Dotto (2006), who observed 64.37 hours, which far exceeds the maximum working hours indicated for Latin American countries, which establishes a working day of eight hours a day and 45 hours a week (PAHO, 2005).

According to studies by Portela, Rotemberg and Waissmann (2005), excessive workload is associated with anxiety, tension, insomnia and lack of time to rest, generating conflicts in household management.

In studies carried out by Girardi and Carvalho (2002) in Brazil, nursing technicians and assistants earn an average of 41.9 per cent of nurses' salaries. In our study, we found that the average salary of mid-level nursing professionals who attend to women during labour and childbirth corresponds to 28.6% of the average salary of nurses, a result very close to that found by Dotto (2006) among nursing professionals who attend childbirth in Rio Branco institutions, corresponding to 33.7% of the salary of nurses, and by Cagnin (2008), who found in Araraquara an average of 39.3% corresponding to the average salary of mid-level professionals in relation to the salary of nurses.

When comparing the institutions involved in this study, we realised that there is a big difference between the salaries of nursing professionals; they show us a different reality, despite the fact that the averages show a level playing field between the classes. The nursing assistants and technicians at the "luz" maternity hospital are paid 18 per cent more than the nurses and obstetric nurses at the lua maternity hospital. This is due to the way they are employed, whereby municipal civil servants receive higher salaries and work shorter hours.

With regard to participation in scientific events, we observed that the professionals studied have little participation in the area of women's health. The data shows that in the "light" maternity hospital, the professionals have 76.6% more participation than the professionals in the "sun" and "moon" maternity hospitals. The reality found was similar to that found in studies on the profile of professionals who provide care to pregnant women, women in labour and puerperal women in institutions in Rio Branco, Acre (DOTTO, 2006) and in the interior of São Paulo, in Sorocaba (GARDENAL, 2002).

In a study carried out by Urbano (2002) on participation in scientific events in the professional field, it was noted that we are at a time of rapid changes in technology and knowledge, which means that we have to seek updates from other sources, such as seminars, congresses, conferences and computerised sources.

The practice of training activities is fundamental for improving the quality of nursing care, as the nursing team is made up of heterogeneous professionals, mainly due to the number of years studied (DAVIM, et aL, 1999).

We noticed in our study, by analysing the nursing professionals, that not all maternity hospitals in the city of Londrina fully meet the definition of a qualified professional set out by the International Confederation of Midwives, the International Federation of Gynaecology and Obstetrics and the World Health Organisation (WHO, 2004b). Although eight nurses (61.5%) meet this profile, when we analyse each institution, we see that in the "luz" maternity hospital, all the nurses specialise in obstetrics, which is not the case in the other two institutions.

According to studies by Starrs (1998), the staff qualified to attend labour and birth can be a professional midwife, a nurse with a specialisation in obstetrics or a doctor with specific expertise and experience.

The professional qualification of nurses is important so that they can keep up with technological advances and changes in society, in order to improve the care provided to clients and act in a critical and reflective manner in the professional sphere (ONOFRE et al, 1990).

In our country, the professionals legally qualified to carry out childbirth are doctors, nurses, obstetric nurses and midwives. It is worth remembering that nurses who do not specialise in obstetrics are only professionally qualified to deliver babies without dystocia, episiotomy or episiorraphy, as regulated by Decree 94.406 of 8 June 1987, which regulates Law 7.498 of 25 June 1986, which provides for the professional practice of nurses and professionals who hold a diploma or specialisation in obstetrics or obstetric nursing (BRASIL, 2002).

Some of the activities carried out by the nurses taking part in this study are not regulated by current legislation in Brazil, such as the use of oxytocin at some point during labour. All the nurses also reported performing episiotomies, episiorraphy and using local anaesthetics.

In our legislation, COFEN Resolution 317/2007 establishes in Art. 1 that it is a nursing action, when carried out by nurses as part of the healthcare team, to prescribe medication, and in Art. 2° it states that this action will be legally limited through the implementation of Public Health Programmes and routines that have been approved in public or private healthcare institutions. In the institutions participating in this study, there is no care protocol that regulates the nurse's actions in terms of requesting the administration of medication. Therefore, these professionals carry out procedures without legal backing.

If we compare the actions regulated internationally, we see that the Core Competencies for the Basic Practice of Midwifery, according to the International Confederation of Midwives (ICM), advocate basic and additional skills for professionals who provide care during labour and birth (INTERNATIONAL CONFEDERATION OF MIDWIVES, 2002). Among the essential competences, we highlight the performance of episiotomy and episiorraphy and the active management of the third period with the administration of oxytocin, which are classified as recommended skills for qualified care (INTERNATIONAL CONFEDERATION OF MIDWIVES, 2002).

Another relevant fact is that all births carried out by nurses are recorded on the hospital admission note (AIH) as a medical procedure, an activity that is contrary to Brazilian legislation, which regulates the performance of normal births without dystocia by obstetric nurses, including the issuing of AIHs. We believe that this is due to the nurses' lack of organisation in drawing up a protocol to ensure their actions in childbirth care. In these institutions, even if the nurses assist with the delivery, it is characterised as a medical procedure, resulting in ethical and legal issues, as they are legally responsible for a procedure that they did not actually carry out.

The World Health Organisation considers that, due to the less interventionist characteristics of their care, nurses are the professionals best suited to caring for women during pregnancy and childbirth. It believes that nurses are the least expensive and most effective professionals for achieving safe motherhood, which contributes to reducing maternal and neonatal morbidity and mortality and the costs of caring for women in the pregnancy-puerperium cycle.

The Brazilian government has tried to encourage the training of human resources, including obstetric nurses, in order to reverse the country's high maternal and neonatal morbidity and mortality rate by qualifying the staff who care for women and their newborns, and has published measures to value the role of obstetric nurses in childbirth care, by means of Ordinances, especially when it included deliveries carried out by obstetric nurses in the SUS payment table, and when it included the group of procedures for Normal Deliveries without Dystocia carried out by Obstetric Nurses in the Table of the Hospital Information System of the Unified Health System (SIH/SUS) and in the Table of Outpatient Information Systems (SAI/SUS), and approved the Nursing Report for issuing Hospital Admission Authorisations.

Therefore, we believe that nurses, in addition to incorporating the recommendations related to professional training, must have active participation and the desire to become an agent of change towards a more humane, less interventionist model of obstetric and neonatal care, based on best practices and scientific evidence. In this sense, concern about the quality of teaching and the training of nurses in the care of women throughout the reproductive period is a priority if we are really interested in helping to reduce maternal and neonatal morbidity and mortality, reduce the high rates of caesarean sections, which are often unnecessary, and change the model of obstetric care in our country.

5.2 Care during labour and childbirth: description of what was observed

In order to define health policies, it is important to assess the competences of the team of health professionals. It is also of the utmost importance to evaluate organisational performance, manage health risks and assess the effectiveness of professional training and education programmes (KAK; BURKHALTER; COOPER, 2001).

In order to provide quality care, health professionals need to master a large number of competences. The assessment of these competences should be planned to cover high-risk or critical areas (KAK; BURKHALTER; COOPER, 2001).

The model of care provided by nurses in obstetrics should be focused on humanising their practices, including social, cultural and economic actions that should include care for women, children and families (SILVA, et al., 2005).

It was possible to observe that there are differences in the care model adopted by the institutions that provide childbirth care in the city of Londrina. We noticed that only the "luz" maternity hospital prioritises professional qualification when carrying out activities with women in labour and childbirth, unlike the other institutions, where nurses play an extremely bureaucratic and unhelpful role, which contradicts the qualified care model encouraged by the WHO.

The presence of a carer is not routinely allowed in the institutions studied in Londrina. We realised that in the "moon" and "sun" maternity wards, this practice is not encouraged at all, unlike the "light" maternity ward, where the companion is encouraged to remain by the parturient's side until the birth. During our observations, we noticed that patients who were accompanied during their pre-natal and delivery periods became more tolerant and less anxious as labour and delivery progressed, because they felt safer and less lonely.

In our country, we have Law No. 11.108 of 7 April 2005, which makes it compulsory for SUS health services and supplementary health services to allow the presence of a companion chosen by the parturient during the entire period of labour, delivery and immediate postpartum. A study by Costa (2004) found that 65.3% of Brazilian municipalities do not allow the presence of a companion during labour and childbirth. We would point out that the law's validity does not guarantee its implementation, and that it requires a process of organising services and professionals to absorb this practice (BRÚGGEMANN; OSSIS; PARPINELLY, 2007). As Schneider (2008) points out, humanised conditions are necessary for welcoming companions, including a suitable place for meals, hygiene and comfort.

Despite the benefits of this practice and the legislation in force, what can be observed is the lack of preparation on the part of professionals to deal with the figure of the accompanying person/father as someone participating in the birth process. On the other hand, it is known that changes in the structure and process of work create new needs. In this specific case, where another element is included in the parturition process, it creates new demands for the parturient and the profcssionals. Therefore, the institutional role is very important in adopting practices that facilitate a paradigm shift in labour and birth care towards more humanised care. However, much progress has yet to be made in adopting these practices, so as not to discriminate or make the presence of a companion dependent on the type of labour or any other prerequisite.

The concept of humanised care is broad and involves a set of knowledge, practices and attitudes aimed at promoting healthy labour and birth and preventing maternal morbidity and mortality, seeking to ensure that the health team carries out beneficial procedures and avoids unnecessary interventions. The Ministry of Health (BRAZIL, 2001) sets out some important actions in caring for women during the pregnancy and puerperal period, and identifying the history of the parturient woman is essential for her admission. The Ministry of Health states that a complete survey of the information contained in the prenatal card should be carried out and possible complications in labour and delivery identified, thus individualising care. It is the health professional's duty to welcome the woman and her newborn with dignity, establish a bond and explain the various meanings of pregnancy for the woman and her family (BRASIL, 2005).

When welcoming women, the professional must be able to receive them from the moment they arrive at the health centre, listening to their complaints and anxieties and providing comprehensive care, ensuring that there is ample coordination with other services (BRASIL, 2005). In our study, we realised that this practice is carried out by mid-level professionals, who carry out low-complexity activities, leaving the more complex procedures to the doctor. It is worth noting that in our findings, we found that checking the pregnant woman's personal details on the antenatal card and identifying the professional who does the welcoming is not part of the service.

We didn't see any nursing consultations carried out by nurses or obstetric nurses, as required by Brazilian law. A similar finding was made by Dotto (2006) in the municipality of Rio Branco/AC, by Cagnin (2008) in the municipality of Araraquara/SP and by Fornazari (2009) in the municipality of Piracicaba/SP (2009).

According to Witt (2005), the main recommendation for reducing maternal and neonatal morbidity and mortality is that all women should be cared for by qualified staff. The importance of nursing work, expressed in the recognition that nurses have a fundamental role to play in the performance of essential public health functions, has been recognised in Brazil by managers and the population; the doubt remains with nurses, because they do not act in their proper spaces (WITT, 2005).

One of the greatest challenges of modern obstetrics is to ensure quality care for women giving birth. The revival of the humanisation and naturalisation of childbirth gained momentum with the Safe Motherhood Project in 1996, when the World Health Organisation (WHO) established strategies to ensure safe practices in pregnancy and childbirth care, publishing practical guidelines for the care of women during the pregnancy-puerperium cycle. In one of these publications, the WHO makes a careful review of the practices currently adopted in childbirth, classifying them into four categories: practices that have been shown to be useful and should be encouraged; practices that are clearly harmful or ineffective and should be eliminated; practices for which there is no clear evidence; and practices that are frequently used inappropriately.

In our study, we found that some of the practices adopted in the maternity hospitals studied in Londrina were in line with WHO recommendations. Trichotomy and enema, practices considered harmful, were not observed as routine practices in the institutions studied. Women should receive impartial guidance on these practices during prenatal care and make a conscious choice about whether or not to perform them (BRASIL, 2001). Contrary to WHO recommendations, there are still institutions in Brazil that perform it routinely (REIS; PATRÍCIO, 2005).

Prepartum bowel preparation was introduced into obstetric practice with the supposed benefit that it would facilitate the descent of the fetal head, stimulate contractions and thus shorten labour; there would also be a reduction in contamination at the time of delivery, minimising the risks of infection for mother and baby. However, scientific evidence shows that its routine use is not beneficial for the couple. In a study carried out on faecal contamination during the evolution of labour and delivery, it was observed that there was no increase in genital infections, nor a decrease in the duration of labour and delivery, and there was no difference between pregnant women of different births (LOPES et al, 2001). However, many services still continue to use it habitually.

Another important issue regarding support during labour is feeding the parturient woman. The WHO (2001) recommends that parturients in labour be offered food and have access to hydration. High-calorie, easily digestible liquids should be offered. Labour can take hours and the expulsion period requires physical effort. Because of these factors, women in labour need to stay hydrated and fed. Fluid intake is also important because it prevents dehydration. However, the belief in restricting and stopping food, solid or liquid, after the start of labour is widely accepted in hospital institutions today.

We observed in our study that the offer of liquids and food is only encouraged in the "light" maternity ward, where liquids (tea and water) and soups are offered, and is only suspended when a caesarean section is indicated.

Compulsory starvation can be a very unpleasant experience, aggravated by the effort of labour, which can be compared to the effort of continuous moderate exercise. Forced fasting can lead to unsatisfactory progress in labour, a diagnosis of dystocia and a cascade of interventions culminating in a caesarean section (ENKIN et al., 2005).

Health professionals must take into account respect for the parturient woman's autonomy, and favouring better physical and emotional conditions during labour necessarily involves re-evaluating restrictive eating behaviours during the process.

Another aspect related to humanised care during childbirth is encouraging walking. According to studies by Oliveira et al (2008), freedom of movement favours fetal descent and reduces the perception of pain; as a result, there is less intervention in correcting uterine dynamics and less need to use pharmacological methods for pain relief. Our findings show that the practice is only encouraged in the "light" maternity unit, by the team of nursing professionals.

Mamede (2005), in her study on the influence of ambulation during labour, observed that even though parturients were free to lie down whenever they wanted, they showed great potential for adherence to ambulation. The author emphasises that many women would move around if they were allowed to do so by the institution, but would only do so if they were instructed or encouraged to try standing or walking. The author goes on to say that in environments where women are

encouraged to move around. When there are structural conditions for this, such as physical space and furniture layout, parturient women end up using
various positions that involve movement, including walking, bathing, kneeling, among others.

The relaxation bath is also a measure to humanise women in labour. Davim et al. (2008) state that the bath is a comfort measure for the parturient woman, as it provides pain relief without interfering with the progression of labour. We realised that the relaxation bath is a routine practice in the "luz" maternity hospital. There is therefore a need for this practice to be more encouraged during the care provided in the maternity hospitals studied.

The most frequently observed procedures during admission were vaginal touch (176%), blood pressure measurement (100%) and auscultation of the fetal heartbeat (91.30%). We would highlight the fact that uterine dynamics were not carried out in all cases (16.30%). Uterine dynamics are essential for assessing the diagnosis and progress of labour. It should be carried out for 10 minutes and take into account the frequency and intensity of contractions.

It is worth emphasising that all the institutions in this study have a cardiotocograph. This equipment is often used incorrectly, only to visualise uterine dynamics in print. Santos (2000) states in his study that cardiotocography is the analysis of the repercussions of uterine contractions on the fetal heart rate (FHR), and is indicated for complications and pathologies that imply a lack of oxygenation for the foetus.

We observed that the auscultation of the BCF and vaginal touch were incomplete, as there was no description of the location or rhythm of the BCF; no notes showed an assessment of the pelvis when performing vaginal touch, a fact observed in all the institutions surveyed. This observation was similar to that found by Dotto (2006) in the municipality of Rio Branco/AC and Cagnin (2008) in the municipality of Araraquara/SP.

Risk assessment is not a one-off activity, but an ongoing procedure that should be adopted during pregnancy, labour and delivery through careful monitoring. This should take into account the physical and emotional conditions of the parturient woman, as well as fetal vitality, the progress of the pregnancy and labour, in such a way as to enable early identification of any signs of risk, with timely referral to more complex services (BRASIL, 2008).

The primary objective of a risk classification is to group women into different categories, for which specific actions can be planned, recommended and implemented. Various classification systems have been proposed, in which a woman's supposed risk factors are identified and added together to produce a total score (ENKIN, 2005). Some classification systems require women to be assessed only once, while others may require reassessment at each antenatal visit. Re-evaluation allows the score to be revised upwards or downwards, depending on the situation (ENKIN, 2005).

Thus, the moment a woman is admitted is extremely important in the context of the course of pregnancy events. A parturient woman who has undergone a risk classification process that is well conducted during prenatal care, by receiving good attention at the time of her admission, can reveal to the professional who is assisting her the possible risks that would direct the behaviour to be taken. In the same way, another parturient woman, even if she didn't receive the best care during prenatal care, at the time of her admission, can be assessed by the professional caring for her and her risk determined, which can influence the course of harmful events, however small the need or opportunity.

Almost as important as the assessment on admission of the parturient woman is the assessment of the progression of labour and its recording. There are various ways of recording measurements of this progress. Most institutions around the world use the partogram. This is a graphic record of dilation and descent of the presentation in relation to time, with an alert line, reached when dilation is less than 1cm per hour, and an action line, which is reached if the delay in progression persists for more than 4 hours. It also allows other controls to be recorded, such as BCF and uterine dynamics, as well as interventions such as drug administration and amniotomy (ENKIN, 2005; BRASIL, 2008).

The use of the partogram provides greater security in monitoring the progress of labour, allowing visualisation of the absence of progression (ENKIN, 2005; BRASIL, 2008). According to the Ministry of Health, the partogram, in addition to being a graphic representation of the progress of labour, is an instrument that serves to document and diagnose alterations and indicate the appropriate conduct to correct deviations, as well as to avoid unnecessary interventions. Since 1994, the WHO has made it compulsory to use a partogram in maternity wards (BRASIL, 2003).

This study reveals that the partogram is only adopted as a routine practice in the "luz" maternity hospital, with most of the notes being recorded by medical professionals. We believe that it is important to raise awareness among professionals who assist women in labour about the importance and benefits of this tool for their care, rather than enforcing it.

Early amniotomy is an intervention traditionally used on the grounds that it has the effect of reducing labour time. Several randomised studies suggest a reduction in labour time of between 60 and 120 minutes. However, it is not yet possible to conclude that early amniotomy has a clear advantage over expectant management, or the other way round. Therefore, in normal labour there should be a valid reason for interfering with the spontaneous process of rupture of the membranes. In this study, amniotomy was performed in only 12 (13 per cent) of the births observed.

Among the different regional analgesia techniques (epidural, caudal, paracervical, spinal), epidural is the most widely used method in labour. It provides better and longer-lasting pain relief than systemic agents (WHO, 2000). According to the Ministry of Health (BRASIL, 2001), epidural analgesia provides pain relief that is considered good by 80 to 90 per cent of parturients. The adoption of epidural analgesia in obstetric care makes intensive use of resources and requires several important conditions: labour must take place in a well-equipped hospital, the technical apparatus must be sufficient, there must always be an anaesthetist available and it requires expert and constant supervision of the parturient. For this reason, epidural analgesia is one of the most striking examples of the medicalisation of normal childbirth, transforming a physiological event into a medical procedure (WHO, 1996). In this study, epidural analgesia was not used in the births observed in the institutions participating in the study.

With regard to monitoring the parturient woman's physical wellbeing during labour, blood pressure is a procedure that is highly valued, although in our findings blood pressure checks were not routinely carried out during the antepartum and immediate postpartum periods. Although it was carried out on all pregnant women on admission (100%), only 40.21% had their blood pressure checked during labour and 44.82% in the immediate postpartum period . Measuring blood pressure makes it possible to assess maternal health conditions. This fact is evident in the practice of the three institutions surveyed.

In our country, hypertensive diseases represent the main cause of direct maternal death among all categories of race and colour (BRASIL, 2009). In a study carried out by Viggiano et al. (2004), pregnancy-related hypertensive disorders were responsible for 57.7 per cent of transfers of pregnant, parturient or puerperal women to the intensive care unit in a tertiary hospital.

To speed up labour, intravenous infusion of oxytocin has traditionally been used, although according to the WHO (1996), as a general rule, oxytocin should be used to correct the dynamics of labour in situations where there is immediate access to caesarean section. In this study, we noted that prescribing and administering oxytocin is not part of the practice of obstetric nurses. All the prescriptions were made by medical professionals, with a total of 45 (48.9 per cent) indications. Health professionals, especially doctors, should be aware that the routine infusion of oxytocin not only interferes with the physiology of labour, but also restricts the woman's movements and, in many studies, women have associated its use with a more painful experience of labour (WHO, 1996).

One way of humanising childbirth care is to allow women to choose their own birthing position. The woman should be advised of the beneficial effects of each position and choose the one that is most comfortable for her. Deliveries in the vertical and horizontal positions allow women to participate actively in the birthing process, as they are less interventionist (GAYESKI and BRÚGGEMANN, 2009).

We observed in this study that the lithotomy position was used in almost all of the deliveries carried out in the institutions surveyed, without them being able to choose. We found that four deliveries were carried out in bed, in the "luz" maternity hospital, at the option of the obstetric nurse. Fornazari (2009) also found that the lithotomy position is routinely adopted for all parturients in maternity hospitals in Piracicaba/SP.

We found that the pressure used on the uterine fundus in the second clinical period of labour, known as the Kristeller Manoeuvre, was a practice used exclusively by the nursing team, with the aim of speeding up the expulsive period of labour. There is no scientific evidence to support its use, as it can cause damage to the uterus, perineum and foetus; therefore, it should be abolished from care (WHO, 1996).

We found that episiotomy is not part of the practice of the obstetric nurses taking part in this study, which is different to the reality found by Cagnin (2008) in the municipality of Araraquara/SP, where episiotomy was performed in 100% of deliveries assisted by nurses, and by Dotto (2006) in the municipality of Rio Branco/AC, where it was performed in 90.9% of deliveries carried out by the nursing team. The WHO classifies episiotomy as a practice that is frequently used inappropriately, and is recommended to avoid third-degree laceration, insufficient labour progression and foetal distress (WHO, 1996).

The International Confederation of Midwives (ICM) and the International Federation of Gynaecology and Obstetrics (FIGO) recommend active management of the third stage of labour. Oxytocin administration, clamping, early cutting and controlled umbilical cord traction are recommended to reduce uterine atony and postpartum haemorrhage rates (INTERNATIONAL CONFEDERATION OF MIDWIVES, 2002).

In our study, we observed that the care provided to parturients in the fourth clinical period of labour is the responsibility of the nursing team. We found that, in the institutions studied, the fourth period begins after dehydration and that the care provided to the puerperal woman is limited to keeping her in the delivery room or in bed. Care consists of assessing uterine involution and vaginal bleeding. Blood pressure is not always measured during this period, observed in only 26 (44.86 per cent) puerperal women.

It is worth remembering that the immediate postpartum period is marked by great maternal risk, and uterine involution, vaginal bleeding and blood pressure measurements should be assessed (WHO, 1996).

We observed in this study that the reception of the newborn is the responsibility of the nursing team and the paediatrician on duty. The nurse assists the paediatrician with initial care and the mid-level professionals are responsible for identifying, bathing and measuring the newborn.

In this research, we were able to identify that the care model provided to parturient women in the municipality of Londrina is focused on institutionalised care and is geared towards the medical model. Our findings are similar to the model found by Dotto (2006) in the municipality of Rio Branco/AC.

Petterson and Stone (2004) defined the Brazilian model of maternal health care services as institutionalised and with limited action by non-medical professionals. In our country, 80 per cent of births are carried out by doctors.

The medical model is characterised by high rates of caesarean deliveries. The rate of surgical deliveries in the maternity hospitals studied was 36.95%, representing a rate higher than the 15% recommended by the World Health Organisation.

The presence of an obstetric nurse in the institutions studied does not guarantee that they provide assistance during labour and delivery. We observed that they carry out many administrative procedures and do not participate in care during admission, labour and delivery. The "moon" and "sun" maternity hospitals do not prioritise the professional qualification of nurses to assist women in labour and childbirth.

We believe that a model of birth care that favours physiology, avoids unnecessary interventions, promotes the inclusion of qualified professionals, in short, that creates conditions for a safe, healthy and meaningful birth, is one option for a model to help reduce maternal mortality.

CHAPTER 6

The analysis of data collected through structured interviews with nursing professionals and non-participant observation of the care provided by them during their actions in childbirth care in the municipality of Londrina/PR allows us to reach the following conclusions:

a) The nursing team involved in labour and birth care in the municipality of Londrina is made up of obstetric nurses, nurses, nursing technicians and assistants;

b) The nursing team was female (100 per cent), with an average age of 38.1 years and stable marital status (68.3 per cent). The average workload was 64.25 hours, above the average found in Brazil;

c) There are differences in the quality of nursing care provided in the institutions participating in this study; therefore, we cannot say that the care provided in the municipality meets WHO and Ministry of Health standards regarding the quality of care provided;

d) There is a predominance of the medical model for childbirth care; the nurse most often takes on a bureaucratic role and plays little part in care activities;

e) Many essential skills for labour and delivery care are not developed;

f) Institutions need incentives to implement actions based on up-to-date evidence.

The results show that the care provided by nurses is in need of the implementation of care protocols, with the aim of adapting care for women during reception, labour, childbirth and the immediate postpartum period.

The work of mid-level professionals is highlighted, but with timid humanisation actions. Obstetric nurse practitioners are limited to just one institution, and even then only modestly.

Many essential midwifery skills for quality care, recommended by the World Health Organisation and the International Confederation of Midwives, are not being fully performed, which reveals a need to implement professional training, thus improving both the training and the performance of these professionals, and thus achieving safe motherhood.

REFERENCES

BRAZIL. Ministry of Health. **Prenatal and Birth Humanisation Programme.** Brasilia. MS, 2000.

BRAZIL. Ministry of Health. Secretariat for Health Policies. Women's Health Technical Area. **Childbirth, abortion and the puerperium: humanised care for women**. Brasília 2001a.

BRAZIL. Ministry of Health. Health Care Secretariat. Department of Programmatic and Strategic Actions. Women's Health Technical Area. **Prenatal and puerperium** care: qualified and humanised care. Brasília: Ministry of Health, 2001b.

BRAZIL. **National Pact for the Reduction of Maternal and Neonatal Mortality.** *Primary care report.* Brasília, year 5, May-June 2004.

BRAZIL. Law n. 7.498, of 25 June 1986. Provides for the regulation of nursing practice and other measures. **Febrasgo Journal.** n. 3, Apr 2002. Available at< http://www.febrasgo.org.br. Accessed on: 15 August 2007.

BRAZIL. National Supplementary Health Agency. The obstetric care model in the Supplementary Health sector in Brazil: scenarios and perspectives. In: Domingues RMSM, Ratto K. M. N. **Favorecendo o parto normal: estratégias baseadas em evidências científicas.** Rio de Janeiro: ANS; 2008. p.27-52.

BRAZIL, Ministry of Health. Health Care Secretariat. Department of Strategic Programme Actions. **Manual for Maternal Mortality Committees.** Brasilia: Ministry of Health, 2009.

BRUGGEMANN, O. M.; PARPINELLI, M. A.; OSIS, M. J. D. Birth support: perceptions of professionals and carers welcomed by the woman. **Revista de Saúde Pública,** São Paulo, v. 41, n.1, p. 44-52, 2007.

CAGNIN, E. R. G. **Nursing care for women in the pregnancy-puerperium cycle:** the reality of Araraquara/SP. Dissertation (Master's in Nursing) - Ribeirão Preto School of Nursing, University of São Paulo, Ribeirão Preto, 2008.

CERANTO, Jacqueline L.T.F; MARTINS, Jeanne I. S; CÚNEO, Joana D arc Pereira. **Quality in nursing care during labour and childbirth.**

Available at: < http://www.uniandrade.edu.br/links/menu3/publicacoes/revista_enfermagem/artigo079.pdf> Accessed on: 04 Nov. 2009.

COSTA, A. A. R. et al, Maternal Mortality in the City of Recife. **Revista Brasileira de Ginecologia e Obstetrícia,** Rio de Janeiro, v. 24, n. 7, p. 455-462, 2002.

DAVIM, R. M. B. et al. Continuing education in nursing: knowledge, activities and barriers encountered in a maternity school. **Revista Latino Americana de Enfermagem,** Ribeirão Preto, v. 7, n. 5, p.43-49, 1999.

DAVIM, R. M. B. et al. Assistance to parturient women by obstetric nurses in the Midwifery Project: an experience report. **Revista Latino Americana de Enfermagem,** Ribeirão Preto, v. 10, n. 5, p. 727-732, 2002.

DOTTO, L M. G. **Qualified childbirth care: the reality of nursing care in Rio Branco-AC**. 2006.148p. Thesis (Doctorate in Nursing) - Ribeirão Preto School of Nursing, University of São Paulo, Ribeirão Preto, 2006.

ENKIN, M. et al. **Guide to effective care in pregnancy and childbirth**. Rio de Janeiro: Guanabara Koogan, 2005.

FEBRASGO. Brazilian Federation of Gynaecology and Obstetrics. Eight steps to safe motherhood. **Basic guide for health services**. Brasília: FEBRASGO/COMIN/OPAS/UNICEF/FNUAP, 1995.

FORNAZARI, D. H. **The role of the nursing team in assisting women during labour, childbirth and the immediate postpartum period in the municipality of Piracicaba/SP. 2009**. 93p. Dissertation (Master's in Nursing) - Ribeirão Preto School of Nursing, University of São Paulo, Ribeirão Preto, 2009.

GARDENAL, C. L. C. et al, Perfil das enfermeiras que atuam na assistência à gestante, parturiente e puérpera, em instituições de Sorocaba/SP. **Revista Latino Americana de Enfermagem**, Ribeirão Preto, v.17, n. 4, p. 478-484, 2002.

GAYESKI, M. E.; BRUGGEMANN, O. M. Perceptions of puerperal women on the experience of giving birth in the vertical and horizontal positions. **Revista Latino Americana de Enfermagem**, Ribeirão Preto, v. 17, n. 2, p. 153-159, 2009.

GIRARDI, S. N.; CARVALHO, C. L. Labour market and regulation of health professions. **Human Resources in Health: politics, development and the labour market**. Campinas: Unicamp, 2002. Chap. 3.2, p. 221-256.

GOMES, F.A.; MAMEDE, M. V.; COSTA-JUNIOR, M. L. Masked maternal deaths: In: BESSA, L. F.; CUNHA,L.A.; FERREIRA, T. F. (Org.) **Saúde da Mulher:** desafios a vencer, Rio Branco. EDUFAC, 2004.

BRAZILIAN INSTITUTE OF GEOGRAPHY AND STATISTICS. Available at:< http://www.ibge.gov.br/cidadesat/default.php. Accessed on 21 September 2008.

INTERNATIONAL CONFEDERATION OF MIDWIVES. **Competencies**. New York: ICM, 2002. Available at:< http://www.internationalmidwives.org>. Accessed on: 10 October 2009.

KAK, N.; BURKHALTER, B; COOPER, M.A. Meansuring the competence of healthcare providers. **Operations Research Issue Paper**. Bethesda, v. 2, July, 2001.

LAURENTI, R.; JORGE, M.H.P.M.; GOTLIEB, S.L.D. Maternal mortality in Brazilian state capitals: some characteristics and estimates of an adjustment factor. **Brazilian Journal of Epidemiology**. São Paulo, v.7, n.4, p 449-60, dec. 2004.

LIMA, V.V. Competência: diferentes abordagens e implicações na formação de profissionais de saúde. Interface-Comunicação, Saúde, Educação, v. 9, n. 17, p. 369 - 79, mar/ago 2005. Available at:< http://www.interface.org.br. Accessed on: 18 Feb. 2009

LONDRINA. MUNICIPALITY OF LONDRINA PLANNING SECRETARIAT: Planning **Directorate. Research and Information Management.** Available at:< www.londrina.pr.qov.br>. Accessed on 25 Aug. 2007.

LOPES, M. H. B. M. et al. The use of enteroclysis in preparation for childbirth: an analysis of its advantages and disadvantages. **Rev. Latino-am Enfermagem**, Ribeirão Preto, v. 9, n. 6, p. 49-55, nov.-dez. 2001.

MACLEAN, G.D. The challenge of preparing and enabling 'skilled attendants' to promote safer childbirth. **Midwifery.** Edinburg. v.19, n.3, p. 163-9, Sep. 2003

MACDONALD, M.; STARRS, A. **Skilled care during childbirth. An information booklet to save women's lives and improve the health of newborns.** New York. n. esp., 2003.

MAMEDE, F. V. **The effect of walking on the active phase of labour.**
2005. 100 f. Thesis (Doctorate in Nursing) - Ribeirão Preto School of Nursing, University of São Paulo, Ribeirão Preto, 2005.

MELLEIRO, M.M.; TRONCHIN, D.M.R.; ANDREONI, S. The caring process from the perspective of nurses at a teaching hospital. In: CIANCIARULLO, T.I; GUALDA, D.M.R.; MELLEIRO, M.M. **Indicadores de Qualidade: uma abordagem perinatal. São** Paulo: icon, 1998. chap. 4, p. 55-77.

MINAYO, M.C.S.; SANCHES.O. Quantitative and qualitative: opposition or complementarity? **Caderno de Saúde Pública,** Rio de Janeiro, v.9, n.3, p. 23962, jul-set.1993.

OLIVEIRA, S. M. J. V.; MIQUILINI, E. C. Frequency and criteria for indicating episiotomy. **Rev. Esc. Enfermagem USP,** São Paulo, v. 39, n. 3, p. 288-95, jul./ago./set. 2005.

WORLD HEALTH ORGANISATION. WHO. **Safe motherhood. Assistance to normal childbirth: a practical guide.** Geneva, WHO, 1996.

PAN-AMERICAN HEALTH ORGANISATION. PAHO. **26ª Pan American Sanitary Conference.** Washington: PAHO, 2002.

ONOFRE, I. et al. A participação do enfermeiro assistencial nos cursos de pós graduação. **Enf. Cient.,** São Paulo, v.10, n. 2, p. 17-22, 1990.

PAN AMERICAN HEALTH ORGANISATION. **Map of childbirth services in the Americas.** Washington: PAHO, 2004.

PAN-AMERICAN HEALTH ORGANISATION. PAHO "Millennium Development Goals - **National Follow-up Report, United Nations,** Brazil, 2004". PAHO/WHO. 2004. Available at:< http://www.opas.org.br/ mostrant.cfm?codigodest=232->. Accessed on 1st June 2010 (a)

PAN-AMERICAN HEALTH ORGANISATION. PAHO **"State of the World's Populations Report, United**

Nations Population Fund", PAHO/WHO. 2004. Available at: http://www.opas.org.br/rh/noticia_det.cfm? idnoticia =224->. Accessed on 1st June 2010 (b)

PAN-AMERICAN HEALTH ORGANISATION. PAHO **"National Pact for the Reduction of Maternal Mortality".** PAHO/WHO. 2004. Available at:< http://www.opas.org.br/mostrant.cfm?codigodest=233-> Accessed on 01 June 2010 (c)

PAN-AMERICAN HEALTH ORGANISATION. PAHO **"Newsletter: Documents".** PAHO/WHO. 2004. Available at:< http://www.opas.org.br/rh/admin/ documentos/Ref_Ed_Brasil.pdf-> Accessed on 01 June 2010 (d).

PAN-AMERICAN HEALTH ORGANISATION. PAHO **"Workstation: Observatory of health workers".** PAHO/WHO. 2004. Available at: http://www.opas.org.br?mostrant.cfm?codigodest=230->. Accessed on 01 June 2010 (e).

PAN-AMERICAN HEALTH ORGANISATION. **Profile of obstetrics/childbirth services in the Americas.** Washington: PAHO, 2004.

PAN AMERICAN HEALTH ORGANISATION. PAHO. **OverView of the nursing workforce in Latin America.** Washington: PAHO/WHO/ICN, 2005. Available at: <http:www. icn.ch/global/Issue6LatinAmericanSP.pdf>. Accessed on: 20. Sep. 2009.

PARANÁ STATE GOVERNMENT. Paraná Health Secretariat. **Health statistics:** Maternal Mortality, 2008. Available at: <http://www. saude.pr.gov.br/Estatisticas/materna/index.html>. Accessed on 25 August 2008.

PEREIRA, M. G. **Epidemiologia - Teoria e Prática.** Rio de Janeiro: Guanabara Koogan, 2003.

PETTERSSON, K. O.; STONE, K. **Profiling midwifery services in the Americas models of childbirth care-a literature review.** Washington: PAHO/WHO, 2004.

POLIT, D. F.; BECK, C.T.; HUNGLER, B.P. **Fundamentals of Nursing Research:** methods, evaluation and utilisation. 5. ed. Porto Alegre: Artmed, 2004.

PORTELA, L. F.; ROTEMBERG, L.; WAISSMANN, W. Health, sleep and lack of time: relations to domestic and paid work in nurses. **Revista de Saúde Pública,** São Paulo, v. 39, n. 5, p. 802-808, 2005.

REIS, A. E.; PATRÍCIO, Z. M. Application of the actions recommended by the Ministry of Health for humanised childbirth in a hospital in Santa Catarina. **Cia. & Saude Coletiva,** Rio de Janeiro, v.10, supL, p. 221-30, Sep.-Dec. 2005.

RICHARDSON, R.J. Pesquisa social: métodos e técnicas. São Paulo: Atlas, 1999.

SANTOS, J. F. K. Assessment of intrapartum foetal vitality. In: NEME, B. **Basic Obstetrics.** São Paulo: Sarvier, 2000. Chap. 23, p.214-217.

SCHNEIDER, D. G. et al. Welcoming the patient and family in the coronary unit. **Revista Texto e Contexo Enfermagem**. Florianópolis, v. 17, n. 1, p. 81-89, 2008

SILVA, L. R. et al. History, achievements and perspectives in the care of women and children. **Revista Texto e Contexto Enfermagem**, Florianópolis, v. 14, n. 4, p. 585593, 2005

SPINDOLA, T.; SANTOS, R. S. Mulher e trabalho: a história de vida de mães trabalhadoras de enfermagem. **Revista Latino-Americana de Enfermagem**, Ribeirão Preto, v.11, n. 5, p. 593-600, 2003.

STARRS, A. **The safe motherhood action agenda: priorities for the next decade.** New York, Family Care International, 1998.

SHIRMER, J. **Overview of specialisation courses funded by the Ministry of Health.** Conference : 15th International Congress on Women's Health Issues/ IV COBEON, São Pedro/Brazil, 2004/CD ROM.

URBANO, L. A. Health reformulations and the new professional profile required. **Rev. Enfermagem da UERJ**, Rio de Janeiro, v. 10, n. 2, p. 142-5, May-Aug. 2002.

TRIVINOS, A.N.S. **Introdução à pesquisa em ciências sociais: a pesquisa qualitativa em educação.** São Paulo: Atlas, 1987.

VIGGIANO, M. B. et al. Intensive care needs in a tertiary public maternity hospital. **Rev. Bras. Ginecol. Obstei,** Rio de Janeiro, v. 26, n. 4, p. 317-23, mai. 2004.

WITT, R. R. **Competences of the nurse in primary care: contribution to the construction of the Essential Functions of Public Health.** PhD thesis, presented to the Ribeirão Preto School of Nursing/USP - area of concentration: Public Health Nursing. Supervisor: Almeida, Maria Cecília Puntel de. Ribeirão Preto, 2005. 336 p.

WORLD HEALTH ORGANISATION. WHO. **Beyond the numbers:** reviewing maternal deaths and complications to make pregnancy safer. Geneva: WHO, 1996.

WORLD HEALTH ORGANISATION. WHO **Reduction of maternity mortality:** a joint. WHO/UNFPA/UNICEF/World Bank statement. Geneva: WHO, 1999.

WORLD HEALTH ORGANISATION. **Managing complications in pregnancy and childbirth: a guide of midwives and doctors.** Geneva: WHO/UNICEF/UNFPA/World Bank, 2000

WORLD HEALTH ORGANISATION. **Maternal Mortality in 2000:** estimates developed by WHO, UNICEF and UNFPA. Geneva: WHO, 2003.

WORLD HEALTH ORGANISATION. **Beyound the numbers: reviewing maternal deaths and complications to make pregnancy safer.** Geneva: WHO, 2004.

ANNEX I

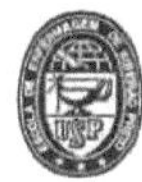 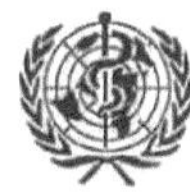 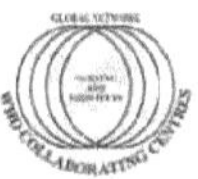

Escola de Enfermagem de Ribeirão Preto - Universidade de São Paulo
Centro Colaborador da Organização Mundial da Saúde para
o Desenvolvimento da Pesquisa em Enfermagem

Avenida Bandeirantes, 3900 - Campus Universitário - Ribeirão Preto - CEP 14040-902 - São Paulo - Brasil
FAX: (55) - 16 - 3633-3271 / TELEFONE: (55) - 16 - 3602-3382

COMITÊ DE ÉTICA EM PESQUISA DA EERP/USP

Of.CEP-EERP/USP – 265/2008

Ribeirão Preto, 05 de dezembro de 2008

Prezada Senhora,

Comunicamos que o projeto de pesquisa, abaixo especificado, foi analisado e considerado **APROVADO AD REFERENDUM** pelo Comitê de Ética em Pesquisa da Escola de Enfermagem de Ribeirão Preto da Universidade de São Paulo, em 05 de dezembro de 2008.

Protocolo: nº 0966/2008

Projeto: PERFIL DA ASSISTÊNCIA DE ENFERMAGEM DURANTE O TRABALHO DE PARTO E PARTO NO MUNICÍPIO DE LONDRINA - PR.

Pesquisadores: Fabiana Villela Mamede
Maria Angélica Motta da Silva Esser

Em atendimento à Resolução 196/96, deverá ser encaminhado ao CEP o relatório final da pesquisa e a publicação de seus resultados, para acompanhamento, bem como comunicada qualquer intercorrência ou a sua interrupção.

Atenciosamente,

Profª Drª Lucila Castanheira Nascimento
Coordenadora do CEP-EERP/USP

Ilma. Sra.
Profª. Drª. Fabiana Villela Mamede
Departamento de Enfermagem Materno-Infantil e Saúde Pública
Escola de Enfermagem de Ribeirão Preto - USP

ANNEX II - INTERVIEW SCRIPT WITH THE NURSING PROFESSIONAL

IDENTIFICATION

1) Gender: ( ) female ( ) male

2) Age: _________________ years

3) Marital status: ( ) single ( ) married ( ) divorced

                 ( ) widowed ( ) consensual union

4) Number of children or other dependents: ______________

5) Remuneration at this institution: __________________

Do you think this remuneration is adequate? ( ) yes ( ) no

If not, how much would the ideal salary be? ___________

6) Do you have more than one job? ( ) yes ( ) no

If so, how many? How many? ____

7) Daily working hours: ____

TRAINING AND PROFESSIONAL ACTIVITY

8) Number of years studied

( ) illiterate   ( ) between eight and eleven years old

( ) between zero and four years old ( ) twelve years old or more

( ) Between four and eight years old

9) Professional training: ____________________________

10) Year completed: _______________________________

11) How did you learn obstetrics (theoretical classes, practical classes, internships)? Where? Total workload? Did you learn to deliver babies? With whom? Was there supervision?

12) Have you taken a postgraduate specialisation course in Obstetric Nursing, with a minimum of 360 hours?

( ) yes ( ) no ( ) in progress

Year: ____ Total workload: ______________hours

13) Is the course funded by the Ministry of Health? ( ) yes ( ) no

14) Have you taken any other specialisation courses?

( ) yes ( ) no ( ) in progress

Which year? _____________________ Year: ____ Total workload: ________

15) Is the course funded by the Ministry of Health?

( ) yes ( ) no

16)   Have you done postgraduate studies?

Master's degree: ( ) yes ( ) no ( ) in progress

Dissertation Name: _________________________________   Year: _______

Doctorate: ( ) yes ( ) no ( ) in progress

Name of Thesis: _________________________________   Year: _______

17)   Did you take any refresher training course(s) in childbirth care after your professional training?

( ) yes ( ) no

Name: _____________________   Workload: _________   Year: ____

18)   Have you taken part in scientific events (in the area of women's health) since your professional training? ( ) yes (

) no

Name: _____________________________________   Year: _______

19)   Have you participated in refresher courses (in the area of women's health) at this institution? (

) yes ( ) no

If not, why not?

( ) institution doesn't offer ( ) no interest ( ) lack of time

( ) Other _____________________________

20)   How long have you worked in childbirth care?

____

21)   Experience with parturients (place and period):

22)   Have you always wanted to work with parturients? ( ) yes ( ) no

23)   Do you enjoy working with parturients? ( ) yes ( ) no

ACTIVITIES CARRIED OUT WITH PARTURIENTS

ADMISSION

24)   Do you check your antenatal card: ( ) yes ( ) no

25)   Do you order laboratory tests? ( ) yes ( ) no

Which ones? _____________________________________

26)   Realise:

Anamnesis ( ) General physical examination ( ) Palpation ( ) Uterine dynamics ( )

Auscultate BCF ( ) Touch ( ) Check BP ( ) Trichotomy ( )

Offer a nightgown ( ) Refer to pre-birth ( ) ( ) Perform enema

Gives a bath ( ) Allows the presence of a carer ( )

27)   Are you responsible for admission? ( ) yes ( ) no

If not, who is the professional responsible? _______________________________

Comments: ____

LABOUR

28)   Do you allow chaperones? What do you do?

( ) yes ( ) no ( ) some of the time. Obs:_______________________________

29)   Do you offer liquids?

( ) yes ( ) no ( ) some of the time. Obs:_______________________________

30)   Do you offer food?

( ) yes ( ) no ( ) some of the time. Obs:_______________________________

31)   Performs/encourages non-pharmacological methods of pain relief:

( ) massage ( ) relaxation techniques ( ) proper breathing

( ) changing position ( ) walking ( ) bathing

( ) Other _______________________________

32)   Do you offer stimulus to pull when dilation is almost complete or complete? ( ) yes ( ) no

33)   Do you use the partogram? ( ) yes ( ) no

If so, when does it start? _______________________________

34)   Do you recommend amniotomy? ( ) yes ( ) no

If so, at what point do you indicate? _______________________________

35)   Do you recommend cardiotocography? ( ) yes ( ) no

If so, at what point do you indicate? _______________________________

36)   Do you recommend administering oxytocin? ( ) yes ( ) no

If so, at what point do you indicate? _______________________________

37)   Does it indicate the administration of drugs for pain control?

( ) yes ( ) no

If so, at what point do you indicate? _______________________________

38)   Do you recommend epidural analgesia? ( ) yes ( ) no

If so, at what point do you indicate? _______________________________

39)   What should be done when identifying foetal distress?

---

40)   Do you recommend caesarean section surgery? ( ) yes ( ) no

If so, at what point do you indicate? _______________________________

PARTY

41)   Do you give birth in this institution? ( ) yes ( ) no

( ) normal without dystocia

( ) normal with dystocia without the help of another professional

( ) normal with dystocia with the help of another professional

( ) twin ( ) pelvic presentation ( ) with meconium fluid

( ) Forceps ( ) assists surgical delivery

42)   Do you allow the woman to choose the birthing position? ( ) yes ( ) no

43)   Do you allow chaperones? ( ) yes ( ) no

44)   Do you offer liquids? ( ) yes ( ) no

45)   Do you recommend administering oxytocin? ( ) yes ( ) no

If so, at what point do you indicate? ____________________________

46)   Do you perform the Kristeller manoeuvre during expulsion? ( ) yes ( ) no

47)   Do you provide perineal protection during expulsion? ( ) yes ( ) no

48)   Do you perform episiotomy? ( ) yes ( ) no

49)   Do you perform controlled umbilical cord traction during dequitation? ( ) yes ( ) no

50)   The moment the cord is clamped:

( ) as soon as the foetus is expelled ( ) after the heartbeat has stopped

51)   Do you examine the placenta and ovular membranes? ( ) yes ( ) no

52)   Uterine revision (manual exploration) after duck? ( ) yes ( ) no

53)   Do you perform episiorraphy? ( ) yes ( ) no

54)   Do you inspect the vagina and cervix for tears?

( ) yes ( ) no

55)   Do you suture lacerations?

( ) 1st grade ( ) 2nd grade ( ) 3rd grade ( ) no

56)   Do you perform local anaesthesia? ( ) yes ( ) no

If yes, when ____

57)   Do you perform regional anaesthesia (pudendal block)? ( ) yes ( ) no

If yes, when ____

58)   Do you provide immediate care for the newborn? ( ) yes ( ) no

If so, which ones? ____

59)   Do you provide immediate care for the newborn? ( ) yes ( ) no

If so, which ones? ____

60)   Mother-child skin-to-skin contact: ( ) first half hour ( ) first hour

( ) second hour ( ) after second hour ( ) didn't happen

61)   Mother/child contact: ( ) first half hour ( ) first hour

( ) second hour ( ) after second hour ( ) didn't happen

62)   Encourages breastfeeding: ( ) first half hour ( ) first hour

( ) second hour ( ) after second hour ( ) didn't happen

IMMEDIATE POSTPARTUM (4TH PERIOD)

63)   Do you check BP? ( ) yes How often? _______________ ( ) no

64)   Do you check uterine consistency? ( ) yes How often? ___________ ( ) no

65)   Do you check uterine height? ( ) yes How often? _______________ ( ) no

66)   Do you check for bleeding? ( ) Yes How often? _______________ ( ) no

67)   Release the puerperal woman to the ward (prescribe discharge from the O.C.)?

( ) yes ( ) no

68)   Do you carry out the nursing evolution at the time of discharge from the O.C.?

( ) yes ( ) no

69)   After how long do you send the puerperal woman to the ward? _______________ h

ANNEX III - INFORMED CONSENT FORM

(Health professionals)

My name is Maria Angélica Motta da Silva Esser, I am a student on the Postgraduate Programme _________ Master's Programme at the School of Nursing of Ribeirão Preto-USP, area of concentration: Public Health. I am carrying out research entitled: **Profile of nursing care during labour and childbirth in the municipality of Londrina-PR,** to obtain a Master's degree in Nursing.

The purpose of this study is to get to know the reality of care during labour and delivery in maternity hospitals in the city of Londrina-PR, with a special focus on nursing staff. To do this, I would like to interview you and observe the actions/interventions you carry out with parturients. This interview will last approximately 30 minutes, and the place and time of the interview will be scheduled according to your possibilities. You will not be identified at any point during the research and you can stop taking part at any time. There will be no cost to any of the parties involved.

I would like to point out that your participation will be very important so that we can find out who the professionals are who work in childbirth care in the maternity hospitals in Londrina-PR, and what activities they carry out.

Thank you for your co-operation, I will leave you a copy of this Free and Informed Consent Form and I am available for any clarifications that may be necessary, by telephone (43) 3328-7349 e-mail: angeluel@hotmail.com, or at my address: Rua Mario Oncken, 300 ap 1403, Jardim das Américas, Londrina-PR.

Thank you.

Maria Angélica Motta da Silva Esser

Having read and understood the information above, I agree to take part in this research and authorise the use of the data for this study, which may be published in scientific events.

Interviewee

ANNEX IV - OBSERVATION SCRIPT: PRE-LABOUR AND CHILDBIRTH.

Number: ______

I. PARTY IDENTIFICATION Date: ______________/ ____ / _____Time: ___

Gesta ـــــ To _______ Abortion _____ Caesarean section ______________ Age:

Gestational age/DUM ___________ Gestational age/USG:______________

Reason: ____

Pre-Christmas: Yes ( ) No ( ) Number of appointments: __ Location: _________

Have you missed any routine examinations: Yes ( ) No ( ) which one? _________

II. ADMISSION Professional who carried out the admission: _____________

Professional responsible for the AIH: __________________________

Identified herself to the parturient ( ) Questioned the complaint at the time ( ) Checked pre-natal card ( ) Checked age ( ) Checked parity ( ) Calculated GA/TA ( ) Calculated GA/US ( )card ( ) Checked age ( ) Checked parity ( ) Calculated GA/TA ( ) Calculated GA/US ( ) Checked routine tests ( ) Questioned obstetric history ( ) Questioned gestational complications ( ) Questioned previous illnesses ( ) Questioned medication use ( ) Questioned smoking ( ) Questioned drug addiction ( ) Questioned alcoholism ( ) Questioned MF ( ) Questioned fluid loss ( ) Questioned bleeding ( ) Performed physical examination ( ) Performed abdominal palpation ( ) Weighed ( ) Checked UA ( ) Checked CA ( ) Checked BP ( ) Checked dynamics ( ) Performed cardiofetal auscultation ( ) Performed vaginal touch ( ) Checked fetal presentation ( ) Checked fetal descent ( ) Performed enema ( ) Checked variety of position ( ) Performed speculum ( ) Offered nightgown ( ) Checked cervical emptying ( ) Checked cervical dilation ( ) Performed trichotomy ( ) Referred to ( ) Had a companion present during the consultation ( ) Explained to the parturient her clinical condition at the time ( ) Discussed the case with the doctor before deciding to hospitalise the parturient ( ) Advised on the next procedures during labour ( )

III. LABOUR

1. Do you offer liquids (food)? Yes ( ) No ( ) Note: _______________

2. Non-invasive and non-pharmacological methods of pain relief:

a) Massage: Yes ( ) No ( ) Note: _________________________

b) Relaxation techniques: Yes ( ) No ( ) Obs: _________________

c) Shower: Yes ( ) No ( ) Note: __________________________

d) Bath: Yes ( ) No ( ) Note: _______________________________________

e) Other techniques: Yes ( ) No ( ) Note: ________________________

3. Use of partogram: Yes ( ) No ( )At what time: _________________

4. Encouragement to walk: Yes ( ) No ( )When: _________________

5. Encouragement to use the ball: Yes ( ) No ( )When: _____________

6. Encouragement to use the horse: Yes ( ) No ( )When: ____________

7. Presence of chaperone: Yes ( ) No ( )What did you do? ____________

8. Identification of foetal distress: Professional: ______________ When: ______

Actions/Interventions: _______________________________________

9. Amniotomy:

Yes ( ) Professional: ___________ When: ________________ No ( )

10. Use of drugs for pain control:

Yes ( ) No ( )Which? ______________________

When: ______________________

11. Use of epidural analgesia: Yes ( ) When: ____________________ No ( )

12. Use of oxytocin: Yes ( ) When? ________________________ No ( )

13. Use of misoprostol: Yes ( ) When: ________________________ No ( )

14. Did you evaluate position variety: Yes ( ) When? ____________ No ( )

15. Did you assess foetal descent: Yes ( ) When? ____________ No ( )

16. Did you assess cervical emptying: Yes ( ) When? ____________ No ( )

17. Did you assess cervical dilation: Yes ( ) When? ____________ No ( )

18. Guided the woman in labour:

Yes ( ) When: ________________________________ No ( )

19. Indication for caesarean section:

Professional: ________________ When: ________________

Reason: ____

IV. LABOUR

Referred time: ____________________ Time of delivery: __________

Obstetric conditions of the parturient: ______________________

20. Professional who realised: ________________________________

21. Was the doctor present: Yes ( ) No ( )

22. The presence of another professional was requested:

Yes ( ) Who? ________________________________ No ( )

23. Place of labour: ____________ Position of the woman in labour: ______

24. Oxytocin administration:

a) during expulsion: Yes ( ) No ( ) b) after discharge: Yes ( ) No ( )

c) at discharge: Yes ( ) No ( )

25.   Presence of chaperone: Yes ( ) What did you do? _________________ No ( )

26.   Does it offer liquid: Yes ( ) No ( ) Note: ______________________

27.   Pull stimulus when dilation is complete or almost complete:

Yes ( ) No ( )

28.   Kristeller manoeuvre during expulsion: Yes ( ) Who did it? __________

No ( )

29.   Protection of the expulsive perineum: Yes ( ) No ( )

30.   Management of the cephalic pole at the time of delivery: Yes ( ) No ( )

31.   Controlled pull of the cord during dehiscence: Yes ( ) No ( )

32.   The moment the cord is clamped:

a) as soon as the foetus is expelled ( ) b) after the heartbeat stops ( )

33.   Examination of placenta and ovular membranes: Yes ( ) No ( )

34.   Mother/child skin-to-skin contact:

a) in the first half hour ( ) b) in the first hour ( ) c) in the second hour ( )

d) after the second hour ( ) e) did not occur ( )

35.   Encouraging breastfeeding: Yes ( ) No ( )

36.   Use of ergometrine after placental delivery: Yes ( ) No ( )

37.   Uterine revision (manual exploration) after childbirth: Yes ( ) No ( )

38.   Did you have an episiotomy: Yes ( ) No ( )

39.   Did you perform anaesthesia before the episiotomy: Yes ( ) Which? __

No ( )

40.   Did you have episiorraphy: Yes ( ) No ( )

41.   Did you perform anaesthesia before episiorraphy: Yes ( ) Which? ___

No ( )

42.   She inspected the vagina and cervix for tears:

Yes ( ) No ( )

43.   Did you suture the lacerations? Yes ( ) No ( )

44.   Did you perform anaesthesia before suturing: Yes ( ) No ( )

45.   NB care: professional ______________________________

What precautions should I take? ______________________________________

V. POST-PARTUM

46.   Have you checked your blood pressure: Yes ( ) No ( )

47.   Did you check uterine consistency: Yes ( ) No ( )

48.   Did you check for involution/uterine height: Yes ( ) No ( )

49. Did you notice bleeding: Yes ( ) No ( )

50. Did you check the appearance of the perineum: Yes ( ) No ( )

51. Time he was taken to the infirmary: _______________________

52. Annotation of the birth in the medical records: professional _____

What was written down? ____

53. Emergency equipment: Yes ( ) No ( )

Who is responsible? ____

VI. OTHER INFORMATION

54. Other actions/interventions carried out:

I) ____

II) ____

55. Emergency situation:

Describe:

Time	PA	Palp.	BCF	DU	Touch	Ocit.	Temp	Profis.	Obser.

Caption: Palp.: Palpation; BCF: Cardiofetal beat; DU: Uterine dynamics; Ocit: Oxytocin; BP: Blood pressure; Temp: Temperature.

ANNEX V - FREE AND INFORMED CONSENT FORM CLARIFIED

(women giving birth)

My name is Maria Angélica Motta da Silva Esser, I am a student on the Postgraduate Programme Master's Programme at the Ribeirão Preto School of Nursing (USP), in the area of concentration: Public Health. I am carrying out research entitled: **Profile of nursing care during labour and childbirth in the municipality of Londrina-PR,** to obtain a Master's degree in Nursing.

The purpose of this study is to get to know the reality of care during labour and delivery in maternity hospitals in the city of Londrina-PR, with a special focus on the nursing staff. To do this, I would like to observe what the nursing staff do and how they do it while you are hospitalised to have your baby. You will not be identified at any point during the research and you can stop taking part without jeopardising your care at this maternity hospital. There will be no cost to you for taking part in the research.

I would like to make it clear that your participation will be very important so that we can identify and describe how childbirth care is being developed in Londrina's maternity hospitals.

Thank you for your co-operation, I will leave you a copy of this Free and Informed Consent Form and I am at your disposal for any clarifications that may be necessary, by telephone (43) 3328-7349 or e-mail: angeluel@hotmail.com, or at my address: Rua Mario Oncken, 300 ap 1403, Jardim das Américas, Londrina-PR.

Thank you.

Maria Angélica Motta da Silva Esser

Having read and understood the information above, I agree to take part in this research and authorise the use of the data for this study, which may be published in scientific events.

Parturient